Mosseri's System for Optimal Health

By Albert Mosséri

Translated by Frédéric Patenaude

About the Author

Frederic Patenaude

Born in 1976, Frederic Patenaude has been working in the natural health movement since his early twenties. He is the author of over 20 books, including *The Raw Secrets,* and his articles are read by tens of thousands of people every week.

Other books & courses from or published by Frederic

For a complete list of available books and products, and to free subscription to Fred's outrageous health and wellness tips, go to: www.fredericpatenaude.com

Your Health is Your Responsibility - IMPORTANT DISCLAIMER

The content, information and recipes in this ebook have been translated and adapted from many books published in French by Albert Mosséri, and other articles, videos and interviews by Frederic Patenaude. The responsibility for the consequences of your use of any methods or techniques described hereafter lies not with the author of this ebook. This ebook is not intended as medical or health advice. No part of this ebook may be reproduced, in any form or by any means, electronic, mechanical, photocopying, or otherwise, without prior written permission from the Frederic Patenaude, www.fredericpatenaude.com.

Introduction to Albert Mosséri and Natural Hygiene

by Frederic Patenaude

Mosséri and Natural Hygiene

In 1996, when I first became interested in the raw food diet and natural hygiene, I came across the writings of Albert Mosséri, an Egyptian-born, French hygienist, who became my main mentor. During his career of 60-plus years in natural hygiene, Mosséri wrote more than 25 books and supervised over 4,000 fasts.

Over the years, I interviewed him and translated some of his material. Mosséri died on February 10th, 2012, at the age of 88.

Long before he died, he gave me rights to his books (as written by Albert Mosséri, in the first person). From them, I created this program.

He really wanted to see this program come to life and hoped that I would publish it, to make his ideas more well-known outside of the French-speaking world.

While others have translated some of his books and materials, this is the first time the complete and priceless information has been translated from the French and edited for readability in English.

This program focuses on his health system. I have not yet translated all of his work about fasting, which may be the topic of a future program.

My Mosséri Interview...and His Life

I had the distinct privilege of finally meeting him in-person in France in 2010, where I sat down for a one-on-one interview at his home in the French countryside, two hours outside Paris. During this interview, Mosséri told me that his interest in natural hygiene began at age 20, when he was still in Egypt. He started by doing research, but I didn't find what he was looking for right away, until he finally found the authors Shelton and Thompson.

At first, he embraced naturopathy, but he gave it up because he felt that it was halfway between medicine and Natural Hygiene.

He started publishing books in his early 20s and when the politics in Egypt took a turn for the worst, he had to emigrate to France where he practiced Natural Hygiene from the start.

But, Natural Hygiene as he practiced it, came in stages—many, many stages. He told me that, "One must find the right diet, the right ideas—and it's not easy to find them. And when we do find them, temptations—external and internal—are so strong that it's not easy to put them into practice right away. It takes years and years to be able to practice pure Natural Hygiene."

My Relationship With Mosséri

If you read my book, *The Raw Secrets*, you're probably aware of this man, who has been a tremendous influence in my thinking and my career. Back in 1996, I discovered raw foods and Natural Hygiene through him—before being acquainted with the raw movement in the United States.

I wrote to him back at the time, and from that we've corresponded on and off until his death.

Mosséri was a disciple of Herbert Shelton. Like Shelton, Mosséri has been a prolific writer, but his books are surprisingly easier to read than are Shelton's. While Shelton writes long, 500+ pages books with dense prose, historical references, and many repetitions to drive in the point home, Mosséri wrote shorter books that read like novels.

In addition to his books, Mosséri published a newsletter that featured French translations of Shelton's work and interesting Q&As with him.

Mosséri has been one of the first hygienists to point out Shelton's mistake of recommending large quantities of nuts daily. For many years, he has warned people against eating too many nuts, seeds, avocados, and oil. Instead, he recommends a diet of fruits, vegetables, steamed vegetables and minimal quantities of fat.

In his career, he's received over 4000 fasters at his former fasting retreat in France. Many of his books have detailed the many fascinating cases he's had to deal with and the lessons he's learned along the way.

In addition to criticizing modern medicine and offering a rational approach to health, Mosséri has also been a strong critic of so-called "alternative medicines", pointing out their fallacies and illogical basis, and explaining why they do not work.

But in spite of his strong stance and belief in Natural Hygiene, Mosséri also had a lot of common sense. He recognized the difficulties that people have applying Natural Hygiene into their lives, and gave practical advice that everybody can use. He was quick to point out the errors that most people make, such as not getting their priorities right and spending too much time in one area of health of little importance, while neglecting the really important ones.

With his permission, I have translated his works, which have never been translated into English, except by me. I think my readers will appreciate the opportunity to study directly from this giant of Natural Hygiene.

My Path to Natural Hygiene: Seeking Perfect Health

I was born in Cairo, Egypt, in 1925. My parents were Israeli, born in Alep, a city in the Northern part of Syria, near the Turkish border.

During my childhood, I was given cod liver oil, like many children of my time. It was supposed to strengthen the body. Apart from this, I rarely took a drug.

In my family, it wasn't common to call the doctor for a simple fever. My mother would put us on vegetable broth until the fever subsided.

Around the age of 12, I had kidney stones. It was a violent crisis that lasted several hours, during which the acute pain made me convulse in my bed, where I couldn't stay still. My mom, seeing the violence of the crisis, called Professor Dunez of the French Hospital of Cairo, who was reputed doctor. At that point, it was something other than a simple fever.

The luminary professor auscultated me and didn't prescribe me any drug. What a chance!. I was put on vegetable broth for a few days and the kidney stones passed without problems.

Fevers and colds were treated without drugs, and antibiotics were unknown at that time.

I finished my Egyptian college degree without problems, late nights and the minimum of study time that my health allowed. I entered Polytechnic University at the age of 18.

My Diet Growing Up

Because I inherited a weak constitution and a very poor vitality, my parents, with the best of intentions, pushed me to overeat. "Eat to strengthen yourself," they repeated constantly.

And so I stuffed myself with bread, five times a day, like every student of my age. My brothers and sisters, who were less gifted than me, followed their instinct and ate according to their hunger, and never overate. My intelligence didn't serve me well in that area.

Here's more or less the menu that my mom gave me:

BREAKFAST: *Bread, butter, cheese or jam, chocolate milk*
10 a.m.: *A sandwich*
LUNCH: *Typical meal including bread, vegetables, rice, and dessert. I hated meat and rarely ate it.*
4 p.m. *A cheese or omelet sandwich*
EVENING: *Almost like noon*

I was never drawn to meat and avoided it. My parents never succeeded in making me swallow a bite of meat, even if it was camouflaged in other foods. I quickly detected it and spit it out. However, I would eat meatballs that were filled with onions and parsley, which masked its horrible taste, thinking it would strengthen me.

I also rarely ate fish but often salami sandwiches, as these sausages had lost their meat taste with all the garlic, pepper and salt they contained.

My Failed Teenage Years

With such a diet, it was no wonder that I couldn't concentrate in school. I had easily explainable digestive troubles and a permanent fatigue, so much that I was forced to abandon my studies to seek a solution to my health problems.

My mind was spacey, and I couldn't concentrate, even just to follow a conversation or a movie. How could I follow high engineering studies that require a sustained mental effort?

Around the age of 18, while wandering in the streets of Cairo, I was drawn by a book in English by Harry Benjamin called *Nature Cure*, along with another one by the same author: *Your Diet in Health and Disease*. I bought the first one, because I was reluctant to make changes in my diet. I was seeking a remedy, but a natural one. I went through the book with an English dictionary, and didn't understand anything, because I knew very little English and my mind was in the clouds. After that, I bought the next book I saw by the same author, and an English magazine called *Health for All*, as well as an American one, *Health Culture*, published every month.

Conscientiously, I read word by word with my dictionary and maybe understood 5% of the content. The articles were never clear and simple. They were too complicated for a young, 20-year old man. Moreover, my mind was clouded by my weak physical condition.

However, I persevered, year after year. I didn't have a Natural Hygiene practitioner to guide me and hold me by the hand towards the perfect health I was seeking. I would surely have gotten there 10 or 20 years sooner.

I had met a naturopath—professor Cohen in Cairo—who pushed me to eat more, due to heat that caused "laziness." I quickly saw he was worthless.

My Failed Trip to London

In 1949, the tragic death of a younger brother gave me courage to go to Scotland, to study with Dr. Thomson at his Naturopathic University. I benefited from the fact that my parent's attention shifted towards this tragedy, to follow my unconventional path. Their hostility to my quest was always great. We had daily fights about it. "Eat like everybody else," they told me relentlessly.

I ate more fruits than my brothers and sisters and my dad, who went to the market every morning, and I didn't buy more than usual. You can only imagine the kinds of admonishments I would get.

This is how I ended up on a plane to London. However, I was denied entry to the country at the border, like many young people for over a hundred years. The overcrowded England always fears the arrival of more immigrants.

However, at the airport I had a short conversation on the phone with James Thomson, who became my first mentor.

My Trip to India

I knew that in India naturopathy was more common due to the English influence. Even Gandhi was a follower, and many fasting retreats were to be found. So I decided to head there.

I arrived in Alwar, a city sitting next to the Himalayan mountains, and stayed there for two months in a palace loaned by the Indian state to be used as a fasting retreat. The place was led by Sharma, a naturopath who was paid by the state for his services.

After that, I headed to Gorakhpur, near Lucknow, north of New Delhi, the capital. There was another fasting center managed by another master Naturopath—Vithal Das Modi—who was 35 years old. When I arrived there, he asked me if I wanted to receive naturopathic care. I told him I was only there to learn. I didn't trust anybody, even though I should have. I wanted to be the one to decide the proper way for treating myself.

I stayed there several months, and during that time the director let me borrow, one at a time, all the English and American books in his library. He had received them in a big box from America, as a gift from a friend.

I read them all, and managed to assimilate a small part of each. But with time, the amount of information that I got gave me a good overview of all the different naturopathic methods.

The type of diet I was served in this center was as follows:

Morning: A piece of fruit
Lunch: Bread, vegetables, salad
Dinner: Same as lunch

In the area, street vendors would sell yogurt in the morning and I would buy that, along with other fruits.

In the afternoons, I would sneak to town, crossing forests and swamps to get there. There were always people sitting there. Once in town, I would wander the streets and stuff myself with yogurt, cakes and Indian sweets. I would come back in a *riksha walla*, a sort of wheeled carriage pulled by a young man. That would cost me one rupiah, which was only a few French francs, for a few kilometers.

How I Embraced Natural Hygiene

My method was to see everywhere I could go and discover what was being done in the Natural Health world. I wanted to read all the books I could in all the languages I knew on this fascinating topic.

I read an Arabic translation from a Russian book on fasting, by an author called *Souvorine*. I read the books of *Dr. Bircher Benner* from Switzerland, *Marchesseau* and *Dextreit* in France, *Harry Benjamin* and *Stanley Lief* in England, and *J.C. Thomson* in Scotland. I also read *Shelton*, and many other American and Spanish authors.

I tried to make a comparison between all the different methods, theories and systems. How could I judge the value of one system without having studied the other ones first? My Cartesian critical mind wanted to be satisfied with all my research. I wanted to know exactly what all these different authors had to say, without ignoring anyone.

Nowadays, it only takes me a few minutes to figure out the content of a naturopathic book, because they're all the same!

The result of this comparative study led me to reject Naturopathy and embrace Natural Hygiene. I consider my main mentors to be *J.C. Thomson* from Scotland and *Dr. H. M. Shelton* from America.

I finally understood that eliminating the cause was sufficient to get results and that all the different naturopathic techniques and modalities are a waste of energy and time. They all seek to mask symptoms, just like traditional medicine. For this reason, I have rejected these methods. My horizon became clearer and so did my thinking.

Upon my return to Egypt, I started to promote Natural Hygiene in French (I am from a French culture), with my books and lectures. A number of French-speaking foreigners lived there at the time and became interested in this new health movement. The movement became quite influential, to the point where a major newspaper published my daily diatribes against traditional methods of healing and presenting the Natural Hygiene methods.

My Move to France

In 1956, the Suez canal became nationalized by Kamal Abdel Nasser, president of Egypt. War broke out involving Egypt, France, England and Israel.

War has never been good to the Natural Hygiene movement, or any green or naturopathic idea. All these different movements for a healthier life become a useless luxury when the life of citizens is in danger and the nation mobilizes itself for a ruthless war.

It was during the Second World War that all healthful living movements stagnated in the Western world. Many of the leaders were sent to the front lines, and all the books and magazines became the last preoccupation of the general public.

In Egypt, war was fatal to the Natural Hygiene movement. Because it was only spread in the foreign communities of the country (French, English, Greek, Spanish, Jewish, Armenian, Iranian and German), Natural Hygiene disappeared when all these foreigners were forced to leave the country and emigrate all over the world. In 1961, I moved to France.

During this troublesome period, while I still lived in Cairo, I was hidden and incognito during months. I owned a factory and the police was looking for me to confiscate it. They didn't find me, as I sold everything and hid away.

On November 21st, 1961, I managed to take the plane and the next day my name was in all the newspapers, in spite of the authorities.

While my parents and siblings emigrated to Israel, Italy, Canada, England, the United States, and Brazil, in an unheard scattering. I chose France, where I landed with my own family. I was met by the police officer Avril, who hosted me at his place.

As soon as I arrived to France, in spite of my residency issues, I launched a movement that spread to Switzerland, Belgium and Canada. I introduced the ideas of Herbert Shelton to the French public.

Why I Wrote This Book

Naturopathy is popular, but Natural Hygiene had a more tangible and lasting impact. However, it's been embraced by only a tiny minority. Very few followers know that Natural Hygiene can be used in cases of catastrophic illness. But many don't have the courage to try it, so they go to the hospital instead.

I've never succeeded in launching a professional Natural Hygienist. They've all been discouraged by the obstacles and difficulties. The very few practitioners that call themselves "hygienists" have turned to

Naturopathy, with their various modalities and a diet that includes so called "organic" bread, meat, salt, honey and wine.

Naturopathic books don't teach much that's useful. Most people, who read these books continue to take drugs, eat meat, smoke and drink wine or coffee. You'll only find recipes and herbal concoctions in these books, and while meat may not be included in the diet plan, there's rarely a strong stance against it. Drugs are rarely criticized, to avoid creating a controversy.

Because they try to appeal to the masses, they've made so many compromises that there's no message left to share. Have they ever healed patients without drugs with natural methods? They rarely come out and say that. They all fear the reprisals by pharmaceutical companies or doctors.

Millions of people sick die every day when they don't need to, and those who know why don't have the right to remain silent. That is why I wrote this book.

Introduction to the Mosséri System

Introduction to the Concept of Natural Hygiene

Once upon a time, there were 100 people with a cold. I have known them all, as you will.

The first one, because he still believed in modern medicine, chose to take a pill.

The second, having been led by his instinct to shun medicines, gulped down a cup of tea with some brandy, according to an old folk remedy.

The third, who only believed in plants (rosemary, borage, etc.) took herbal tea and breathed the pungent steam until she choked.

The fourth, a fitness fanatic bodybuilder, took a cold shower early in the morning.

The fifth took a hot bath with added aromatic plants.

The sixth, a fervent adept of naturopathy, dipped his butt in the cold water of a bidet while pumping his cheeks, and called this 'hydrotherapy'.

The seventh, who swore by spiritual healing, went to receive the magnetic touch of a healer, himself with a cold.

The eighth, who believed in infinitesimal doses, let fall in her mouth a few tiny homeopathic pills.

The ninth, having read somewhere in the newspaper about the discovery of a miraculous vaccine, rushed to his doctor to get immunized, before the vaccine had run out.

The tenth, who had an inclination toward more exotic medicine, went to see an acupuncturist to get the inside of his nose tickled.

The eleventh had tons of tubes of cream in her pocket, which she used to smear her stuffed nose.

The twelfth had a certified chiropractic doctor play with his 33th vertebra, well knowing that there are only 32. And so on.

But, the 100th did nothing to cure his cold. He let Nature do its work, but intelligently. He did not use any remedy, and rested his body and his stomach, skipping a few meals.

The result was staggering and unbelievable at first: all of these persons suffering from a cold, without exception, recovered after some time.

Each and every one got rid of his or her cold, and healed entirely. But the last person, the 100th one who did not use any remedy and who, in all logic, should not have healed this person recovered, too.

So to be clear in my mind about this, I went to question these people, one by one.

- The Advil cured me, declared the first person.
- It was the tea, with added cognac, that cured me, said the second.
- It was the herb tea that cured me, said the third.
- The cold shower cured me, said the fourth. Try it out yourself.
- The warm bath cured me, said the fifth, and so on.

All of these sick people recovered from their colds using different and sometimes contradictory methods, but everyone thought that it was his or her method that was the cure. And everyone could prove it, even the one who had not used any remedy.

Has not medicine also established statistics to prove the efficiency of this drug or that one? This is how we can prove that every remedy—be they contradictory, chemical, or natural—can cure a cold. Aspirin, cold water, hot water, herb teas, cognac, tea, etc., all are effective.

And statistics proving the efficiency of myriad remedies can even be established. But, the most amazing thing is that the sick person who had not used any remedy had recovered, too.

Of course, this is why we must not quickly accept such proofs, testimonials, or statistics, because they do not prove anything at all.

All they prove is that Nature, without being disturbed by this superstitious noise, pursues her work to eliminate the cold and all the other toxins of the other diseases until the person is cured. Even if she must accomplish its work heroically, in spite of all the obstacles put in its way. Even if she ends up frustrated by the energy wasting of the sick and by their demise through fatal diseases.

A cold, like many serious diseases, is a symptom of elimination. But, elimination requires nervous energy. All remedies waste this nervous energy, and in the end, slows down elimination.

In conclusion, most remedies — natural, chemical, or otherwise — have no use. They only hinder nature in its work of elimination. *The sick who recover do so in spite of remedies. They recover much faster when no remedies are used, and Nature is obeyed.* That way, only the rest of the body and of the stomach spare energies and recharge the batteries.

We can neither force the cells to eliminate faster nor to be healthy without eliminating them (as is the hope of allopathy). This elimination must *not* be stopped, because it purifies the body.

An Iranian Man Tells the Story of His Marvelous Recovery

The following is quoted from the book *Raw Eating,* by Aterhov.

"The fact that at age of 60, I am able to write these lines is due to raw-eating.

"Seven or eight years ago my heart was in such poor condition that a heart attack seemed inevitable. I used to get breathless climbing a few steps; I had not strength enough to lift a bucket of water. Constipation, indigestion, heartburn, insomnia, headache, piles, gout, sclerosis, high blood-pressure, tachycardia, chronic bronchitis, hemorrhoids, and frequent colds had been the companions of my life for a long time past.

"Thanks to raw-eating, I have gotten rid of all those disorders. I have permanently lowered my blood pressure dramatically, and my pulse rate went from 80-90 beats per minute to 58-60. Without any sign of fatigue, I can walk to Tajrish and back (a distance of 24 kilometers) in four hours, climb up mountains like a goat, lift heavy suitcases up the staircase and, when I have time, take a stroll of 12 kilometers as an ordinary daily routine. I, who at one time suffered from chronic bronchitis and was laid up with influenza several times a year as a matter of course, have not even had a common cold in the last few years and have slept in the open air all the year round in winter and in summer, without the least fear of either cold or microbes.

"Years ago, I had such a severe attack of gout that I could not touch the joints of my big toe, but today I can twist them with all my might without the least sign of pain. Where in the world have similar results been obtained by means of atophan, ACTH, digitalis, bromides, iodine, aspirin, antibiotics, and thousands of other medicines?

"The heart that works at the rate of 58 beats a minute can be confidently expected to carry on working for a great many years without ever being subject to the danger of a stroke. But with cooked foods, a similar drop in the pulse rate occurs only when the heart is weak, but in my case it is the natural result of the regularity in the operation of my digestive organs.

"It is extremely significant that whenever I try to overload my stomach with several times the normal quantity of natural foods, they do not stay in the stomach for long, but instead, pass into the intestines at once and leave the body in a few hours, without undergoing any decomposition and without producing the slightest digestive disorders or causing me any discomfort whatsoever. Under this condition, my pulse rate is increased by no more than four or five beats a minute, whereas when I try to "satisfy" myself with cooked food like 'an ordinary human being,' my heart beats immediately jump up to 85-90, and it takes days for my stomach to regain its normal feeling of lightness.

"Along with myself, I am bringing up my third child as a raw-eater. She is already a little girl of seven years of age, but she has never put a single morsel of degenerated food into her mouth. Her health is the embodiment of perfection. I can now see what a great difference there is between raw-eating and cooked-eating children. It is easier to bring up a hundred raw-eating children than a single cooked-eating child. I never have the occasion to worry about this child's ailments, such as chills and colds, diarrhea, and constipation, or trouble about the child's eating too much or too little.

"She is as cheerful as a lark and whenever she wishes she goes to the table and helps herself to anything that she likes to eat. She plays, sings and dances all day long without any whims, without crying, without causing trouble to those around her. She goes to bed at exactly 8 o'clock in the evening and, after singing to herself for a few minutes, she closes her eyes and sleeps like a top until 6 o'clock in the morning. Moreover, it is a most remarkable fact that after the first few months we can remember only three or four occasions when she has woken up during the night. So deep and sound is her sleep that no noise or movement causes her to wake up.

"When other children in the kindergarten sit at their breakfast table to have bread and cheese, bread and butter, pastries, etc., she brings out her bag of fruit that she has taken from home and enjoys it quietly. When we are on a visit to friends, she looks with complete indifference at those overloaded tea tables around which people seat themselves and 'enjoy' all kinds of pastries and sweets. Very often she fills the plates of her toy tea set with those sweets and plays 'cooked-eater's tea party' with her dolls and her playmates. She never expresses a wish, not even out of curiosity, to taste any of them. It is in this way that all raw-eating children should be brought up.

"My wife, upon whom I have never forced any of my views, is gradually changing her ways of eating for the sake of her child and her health, and has now become a raw-eater who is quite content with her condition. To begin with, she gave up meat altogether and then she reduced meatless cooked dishes to one or two a week. As the child grew up a little more, these were replaced by a few boiled potatoes taken occasionally. Finally, these too were entirely given up when one day the child asked, 'What is that nasty smell from, Mommy?' After that she took only a thin slice of whole meal bread, which she sometimes ate with honey and walnuts, unseen by the child. Today, she sees the wonderful effect of raw-eating on her organism, and it is not surprising, therefore, that she abstains from all cooked foods. And all this was accomplished without much difficulty, once the decision was made in earnest. When there is no smell of cooked food in the house, raw-eating becomes a very simple matter. This is the way that should be followed by all those parents who value their health and love their children." *(End of quote by Hovanessian)*

Experiences with the Raw Food Diet

I started this book with the story of this man to showcase the benefits of a raw food diet. Because most of the natural health field is influenced by raw food theories, I found it useful to go back to this controversy and evaluate the role of both cooked and raw foods in the human diet.

Before I go on with Hovanessian's story, I wish to clarify something.

According to my experience, people who inherited a strong constitution can overwork themselves and develop heart problems. Weaker individuals can't.

Hovanessian was able to bring down his heart rate from 80 to 60 bpm, another proof of his exceptional heredity, much like athletes who have a resting heart rate of 45 bpm. Some people who don't have such lucks in their genes can't bring down their heart rate below 72 and will not be able to walk 15 miles a day, even while following a raw food diet.

On a raw food diet, there's little risk of overexertion and heart failure. You will always experience fatigue before the "rupture point" and be forced to rest. On the other hand, a diet of bread and meat, overexertion, and going beyond the limits of the human heart will be more likely.

Note by Frederic:

I first heard of the book "Raw Eating" in Mosséri's books, in 1996. I then came across a book called Nature's First Law, by Dini, Wolfe and Arlin. The authors tried to pass off Hovanessian's work as their own, until the scam was discovered, years later.

It's still a remarkable book full of enthusiasm. Mosséri will start off the next chapter will more quotes from Raw Eating, and right after will present his own thoughts on cooking and the raw food diet.

Can We Live on a Raw Food Diet?

The man in story is the Iranian author by the name of A.T. Hovanessian, who published a surprising book in English on his experiences, called *Raw Eating*: *or A New World Free From Diseases, Vices and Poisons*. **On the cover of this book, we can read the following:**

- The cause of human diseases has finally been discovered: all diseases have a common cause — the introduction of cooked foods and other toxic substances in the organism.

- The only radical way to cure diseases is to eliminate cooked foods and other toxic substances.

- Cooking destroys the nutritional properties of foods and converts them into toxic substances.

- All scientific data regarding the nutritional value of proteins, vitamins and minerals are false.

- The spread of raw foodism represents the most humanitarian and noble world one can do in the 20th century.

I have read the book by Hovanessian—also called Aterhov—and have been greatly impressed by it. However, I cannot agree with all of its conclusions.

- When Hovenassian (Aterhov) says that the cause of human diseases is cooked foods and other toxic substances, we should clarify what these "toxic substances" are. The "toxic substances" refer to chemicals, drugs, alcohol, pesticides, preservatives, spices, but could also extend to stress and its consequences. Those causes are actually much worse than cooked foods for health.

- As we'll see in the next chapter, many healthy people live on a diet of cooked foods and manage to stay in perfect health.

Here are a few select quotes from the book by Hovenassian (Aterhov):

- "Raw vegetable food should be the only nourishment taken by man. The habit of eating cooked food should be abandoned in this world once for all. This is the unerring demand of nature. The consumption of cooked food is the most terrible barbarism in the history of mankind, a barbarism that no one seems to be aware of and to which everybody falls an unconscious victim. No matter how strange the idea may seem to some, it is the absolute truth with which we cannot but agree."

- "Until the discovery of fire, along with the rest of the animal kingdom, man had developed and carried out his evolution by the consumption of natural, raw nourishment. But since the discovery of fire, without much reflection, men have put natural foodstuffs on the fire, have destroyed their essential constituents, have debased them and have then nourished their bodies with them. As a direct consequence, there have resulted all the diseases, from which all mankind suffer today."

- "The human organism is the masterpiece of nature. Man is the most complicated and the most perfect living factory constructed by the unceasing efforts of nature over a period of 1.5 billion years. Simultaneously, with the construction of this factory, our wonderful nature has made use of the rays of the sun to develop all the raw materials which are necessary to coordinate the thousands of complicated operations of our organism and to ensure corresponding production. Furthermore, nature has placed those raw materials in their entire perfection and in the faultless harmony of their various constituents in a tiny grain of the corn, in a pulpy seed of a pomegranate, in a berry of the grape or in a leaf of a plant. Each of the "paltry" foodstuffs taken separately contains all those factors that are necessary to keep alive the living organism of a being like man."

- "In the material world, the smallest deviation from the details developed by an engineer for the smooth working of the mechanism of a factory, or a fault in the raw materials specified to ensure its normal productivity, results in a corresponding breakdown in the operation of the plant. In the same way, the slightest deterioration or alteration in the raw materials prescribed by nature to ensure the smooth operation of the complicated processes of the human organism causes disorders in the normal biological functions of our organs and these disorders appear in the form of diseases."

- "The various methods employed by man in destroying or degenerating the fully-balanced raw materials prescribed by nature for the normal operation of his organism do not bear thinking. For that purpose, civilized man has invented demoniacal factories, ovens, furnaces and kitchens. Every degeneration in the quality of natural foodstuffs is followed by a corresponding degeneration in the human organism. Natural nutrition ensures the normal operation, of our organism, while unnatural nutrition is followed by an abnormal discharge of its functions. The multiplicity of illnesses is the result of the great diversity of degeneration in the constituents of natural foodstuffs."

- "Provided that all its needs are satisfied by the laws of nature, the human organism, which is the most perfect organism in the animal kingdom, can live in excellent health from a minimum of 150 years to a maximum of 200-250 years. Cooked foodstuffs force human organs to work in several times their normal capacity, tire them out prematurely, cause various illnesses and shorten man's life to a fraction of its normal span."

- "The reader may naturally wonder why none of the numerous eminent scientists and professors see these simple truths and why nobody tells us that the habit of eating cooked food is unnatural and dangerous. The reason is that the whole of mankind are food-addicts and food-addiction has blinded everybody. Nobody realizes that cooked-eating is a vice and that it is indeed the most terrible of all vices. It is not a craving after only one kind of substance, but the sum total of one's voracious longings for thousands of substances (and what "marvelous," "desirable" substances at that!). Besides, short-sighted cooked-eaters see richness and excellence in the multiplicity of the debasements to which foodstuffs are subjected, whereas it is that very multiplicity of the debasements that give rise to a multiplicity of harms, the true reflection of which can be seen in the large variety of illnesses that prevail in the world."

The Demand for Cooked Food is Not Hunger

"When a cooked-eater tries to feed on exclusively natural foodstuffs, such as honey, walnuts, grains, raw fruits and vegetables, and he has no further appetite for any sort of raw food, the natural demands of his organism are at that moment completely met and he is satiated. But in spite of this, even if he should have already taken several times his normal daily requirements of foodstuffs, he still behaves as though he had eaten nothing and feels a great demand for a dish of highly-seasoned meat, rich and appetizing. This is not hunger any more. It is the irritation caused by the poisons which have been stored in the body and which now demand fresh poisons. It is the cry of the demon that lies there sprawled and demands new tools to tear the human organism to pieces. The prudent, strong-willed raw-eater hears that cry in all its vehemence day in and day out, but he ignores it with all his soul and does not make one jot of concession."

Cooked Eating Forces the Human Organs to Work at Three to Four Times Their Normal Capacity

"All the human organs have a store of natural reserve energy. Usually, they work at a quarter of their potential capacity, keeping the rest of their energy for later use in a special emergency or during old age. Thus, in "normal" circumstances the pulse rate of the heart is 70-72 beats per minute (while that of a raw-eater is only 58-62), which in exceptional circumstances may be raised to over 200 beats per minute. Again, during normal respiration 500 cc's (or cm^3) of air passes into and out of the lungs, but by a special respiratory effort we can inspire as much as 3700 cc's."

"The raw-eater makes use of his digestive organs at one-quarter their potential capacity, as a result of which his organs are never overloaded or fatigued. The cooked-eater, on the other hand, after stimulating his appetite by means of conditioned reflexes, irritating spices, aperitifs, and other absurd stimulants, fills his stomach to such an extent that the digestive organs are forced to bring into action all their reserve energies and even then they are unable to cope with the demand placed upon them. Whereupon man is forced to return the loathsome food by the same channel as he sent it down or to expel it from his intestines with purgatives. Surprisingly, enough such nauseating acts are not considered strange by a cooked-eater."

"By the overloading of the digestive organs a great many accessory organs are set to work, too, such as the heart, the liver and the kidneys. The additional work performed by these organs soon has the effect of tiring them out and putting them out of action prematurely. It is not surprising, therefore, that as a result one's life is shortened several times. By feeding on useless, harmful and poisonous substances the food-addict gratifies his passions, paralyzes the action of his stomach, and creates for himself the illusion of being satisfied, whereas his cells are, in reality, moaning with hunger for lack of essential nutrients. The stomach of a raw-eater is always at rest, even though it is generally empty, but his body is indeed full and satisfied in the true sense of the word."

Short-Sightedness Is the Greatest Defect of Medical Science

"The greatest mistake of biologists who are addicted to cooked food is their short-sightedness. They close their eyes to those harms that appear small and do not foresee the serious consequences that, sooner or later, result from seemingly negligible causes."

Let us illustrate our statement by a few examples.

"Cooked meals, especially meat dishes, are full of poisons. Now, nobody takes any notice of the chronic poisoning that goes on imperceptibly all the time, and even when, as a result of such poisoning the liver, the heart or the kidneys are damaged in time, the condition is attributed to unknown causes. When the poisoning is still severe and is accompanied with diarrhea and vomiting, it is regarded as a gastric disorder. By poisoning they understand only that condition which affects the whole organism and threatens the victim with immediate death. How many innocent lives are sacrificed in this way?"

"Men do not see the filth that passes into their arteries and veins through the medium of food every day, and when it sits layer after layer on the walls of the vessels, narrows their passages and suddenly stops the circulation of the blood one day, short-sighted people regard the occurrence as "unexpected."

"In the opinion of short-sighted people, raw-eating is tantamount to a return to the primitive life of the prehistoric man. In point of fact, there is no greater disgrace to civilization than the operations of cooking and refining. The raw-eater merely forgoes the miseries caused by the so-called diseases of civilization and refuses to turn the technical progress bestowed upon him by civilization into a means of destroying the purity of the human raw materials. Otherwise, he does not forgo the convenience of speaking by telephone, traveling by plane or keeping his fruit fresh in his refrigerator."

"For centuries, men have been so blind and ignorant that they have always regarded the eating of cooked meals as a natural operation. And now, when for the first time, they hear about raw- eating, they regard it as something strange and curious. Whereas in reality it is precisely the degeneration of natural foodstuffs by means of cooking that is most unnatural, strange and curious, and which must be recorded in history as the greatest folly committed by Homo sapiens."

"I publicly appeal to all scientists, neither to confirm my views and declare them to the whole world nor to prove that when natural foodstuffs are put on the fire no losses are incurred in their nutritive constituents or energy contents. That No deaths occur of the living vegetable cells and no changes take place in the constitution of the atoms. Scientists must further prove that in the creation of nutrients for the human organism our Creator has made a mistake in not presenting them to us with the foodstuffs in a "purified," cooked, or burned state, that the operations carried out in factories and in kitchens are scientific measures aimed at correcting the errors of the Creator and that the artificial vitamins made by man have greater nutritional values than the vitamins found in nature. Failing that, they must admit the tragic mistakes that have been made hitherto and, doing away with cooked meals once for all, they must take refuge in the wisdom of the Creator and stop interfering with the composition of the natural foodstuffs created by Him. Let those who regard themselves as meat-eaters consume their meat, if they can, fresh and entire, like carnivorous beasts do, without killing its cells or degenerating it in any way."

"We have no right to upset the integrity of the raw materials created by nature for the human organism when:

- With all the scientific means at our disposal, we are not able to create the tiniest single-celled organism.

- With the help of all the nutritive constituents known to us, we cannot feed an organism artificially and keep it alive for long.

- We have barely succeeded in recognizing a thousandth part of the substances in a grain of corn."

"It is true that a great deal of research has been carried out and considerable progress has been made on the recognition of various nutrients and as a result many important nutritive constituents have been discovered, but all those discoveries cannot be of greater significance than the invention of artificial satellites. The difference between artificial vitamins and the nutritive constituents composing a grain of corn is of the same order as the difference between man-made artificial satellites and the heavenly bodies forming our whole galactic system. The scientists who make artificial satellites, however, never presume to annihilate the existing galaxies and replace them by heavenly bodies newly created by themselves."

"Our best course is to study carefully the laws of the natural evolution of animal and vegetable organisms, and then to assist the work of nature by using every natural means to speed up that evolution. But, under no circumstance, must we undo the work of nature and then try to reconstruct it by the help of miserable gland extracts and artificial vitamins."

"When we place a piece of potato or marrow in butter and begin to fry it, we start the process of its destruction right from the first moment. It immediately begins to sizzle, to shrivel, to become brown and then to dry up, and if we continue the operation a little longer, it chars up and turns into mean ashes. That appetizing smell which tickles our nostrils is the smell of the most valuable constituents of natural foodstuffs, which laugh at our senses and vanish into thin air."

"The terms "cooking" and "baking" must not be used in the sense of preparing, constructing, and improving, as they have been uses until now. They must be employed, rather, to convey the sense of ruining, destroying, burning, killing, or annihilating, because by those operations we destroy the most valuable substances that are of vital importance to our organism and thus we commit the most heinous crime against humanity."

"By the victory of raw-eating, lasting peace will be finally established in the world and cooperation will be set up between nations. All crimes, hatred, enmity, arrogance, jealousy, and, in general, all the evil habits and beastly inclinations of man are the offspring of cooked-eating. By the abolition of cooked-eating the passions of men will calm down, their minds will be ennobled, and life will become so easy that men will no longer be obliged to tear each other's flesh or sell their conscience for a mess of pottage."

—END OF QUOTES—

I quoted quite a bit from Aterhov's book, as it's written with such enthusiasm and passion and is in line with Natural Hygiene, except for a few important considerations:

- Cooked foods are certainly not the only, or even the main, cause of human diseases. Aterhov obviously got a little taken away by his own momentum and enthusiasm.

- His work would have been more accurate if he had claimed that "most" human diseases could be avoided through a raw food diet, but not "all diseases."

- Even wild animals eating a raw food diet suffer from some diseases, although less numerous than those of humans.

In the next chapter, we'll discover that it's possible to remain in perfect health eating conservatively cooked foods, while avoiding condiments and the worst forms of cooking like frying.

The Raw Food Diet

The Raw Food Menu

In practical terms, how should we eat according to Hovanessian's diet?

I have summarized his daily menu as follows. All foods are of course eaten raw.

1. Fresh raw fruit.
2. Dried fruits, generally soaked
3. Nuts and seeds, generally ground
4. Daily salad bowl.

The salad he recommends can include:

- Greens
- Other vegetables sliced thinly or grated
- Sprouted grains and beans (lentils, wheat, etc.)
- Raw potatoes, grated
- Raisins, dates, dried figs, soaked the night before
- Nuts and seeds, blended with water to create a dressing
- Honey
- Lemon juice
- Olive oil

Drinks
For children, a bit of honey or lemon juice in a glass of water.

Cakes
Stuff dates or figs with almonds or other nuts, with vanilla, cinnamon or saffron.

Sandwich
Almond butter inside lettuce leaves can make a good sandwich.

Hovanessian's Diet

His diet includes two meals.

1. ***First Meal***: Fresh fruits
2. ***Second Meal:*** a big salad as previously described, seasoned with soaked dried fruits oil and honey.

My Comments on This Diet

Overall, Hovanessian's diet is excellent, but I have two comments:

1. **Smart hygienists avoid honey**. It's an animal product made by bees for the needs of bees, not for people who steal it from them. Eating honey can cause cavities, pinkeye (conjunctivitis), and decalcification. Honey, contrary to common belief, doesn't contain a lot of vitamins and minerals. Often claims are made about honey that are just copied from honey marketers, without any proof. One of my patients, who ate too much honey, experienced hair loss as a result.

2. **Nuts and seeds should be limited**, due to their fat and protein content. I also recommend avoiding oil, although some people find it easier to eat a salad with a bit of olive oil in it — a compromise I'm willing to permit.

Can We Live on Cooked Potatoes?

How to Judge Cooking

After having praised the virtues of raw foods, how should we judge cooking? Is it a very important cause of disease? Exactly where does it fit in the hierarchy of the causes of disease? Should we consider it, as some people do, the main cause of all diseases on Earth?

The discovery of a tribe in perfect health, living somewhere in the mountains in New Guinea, will set our watch straight, so we can avoid errors in judgment. What is this tribe living on? Surprisingly, they live on a diet consisting of 90% cooked sweet potatoes.

My conclusion is that cooking is not the main cause of disease. There's also a difference between different types of cooking.

Certain types of cooking should be avoided, such as cooking at high temperatures, such as are reached in an oven. Frying in butter or oil causes the fat to become denatured and carcinogenic.

I recommend a sort of "half-cooking," done quickly in a minimum of water not going significantly above 100 degrees Celsius.

The Report From Dr. Bircher

Here's an excerpt from the report of Dr. Maximilian Oskar Bircher-Benner, published in "Der Wendepunkt" #10, 1969:

During an expedition in the interior regions of New Guinea, Hipsley and Clement from Sydney, Australia, discovered an indigenous tribe living in the mountains of Mount Hagen at altitudes reaching 1500 and 2200 meters. They lived on the same plant foods year-round, consisting in 80 to 90% of sweet potatoes.

The rest of their diet consisted of young shoots, sugar cane, green vegetables, bananas, heart of palm, nuts and seeds and other similar products.

In spite of this very spartan diet, the entire population, including children and teenagers, were apparently in excellent health and accomplished great feats of physical labor.

Every member of the tribe ate these sweet potatoes cooked on hot rocks, while vegetables were eaten raw. Almost no fat was consumed by the tribe, since the sweet potatoes contains less than 0.2% of fat.

After having read this report, we cannot accuse cooking of being the main cause of the diseases of humanity. We can still speak against frying and other forms of cooking.

It also goes to show that the absurd theory of the "balanced diet" promoted by modern medicine doesn't hold water. This New Guinea tribe ate almost no fat, and very little protein, as we'll see in the next part of the report below:

Professor H.A.P. Oomen, director of the *Tropical Hygiene Institute of Amsterdam*, took an interest in the case of these natives who have subsisted on such basic fare during centuries.

He discovered that their daily consumption of protein was of 9.92 grams, because sweet potatoes contain 0.5 to 1.5%. On the other hand, they eliminated in their feces 15 times more protein than they took in through their diet of sweet potatoes, eating 1.4 to 2 kilos a day.

The natural conclusion was that proteins were synthesized in the body through an unknown process. It was discovered that these men maintained in their intestinal track a strain of bacteria able to fix nitrogen in gaseous form, through synthesis of amino acids, even those that are considered essential.

This ability is not yet explained in all of its phases, but we can assume that it is of great importance, considering the large quantities of protein eliminated through the feces of the tribe members, as well as their excellent physical health. No nutritional deficiencies were observed.

The tribe ate around two kilos of sweet potatoes a day, which equates to a more generous and varied selection of fruits and vegetables.

Sweet potatoes have a similar composition as white potatoes, but are more difficult to digest due to their sugar content.

I also noticed that the authors of the study made a mistake in calculating the protein content of sweet potatoes. 1.4 kilos of sweet potatoes contains a minimum of 7 grams of protein, and a maximum of 21 grams. 2 kilos of sweet potatoes contains a minimum of 10 grams of protein and a maximum of 30 grams.

We should also add the other foods consumed that also contain protein. It's clear that the number of 9.92 quoted in the report was the lowest number possibly attained. The maximum would be 35 grams.

Table Showing Protein Minimum and Maximum
Potatoes (minimum): 1.400 g = 7 g of protein
Other foods: 160 g = 2 g. of protein
-----
9 grams

Potatoes maximum: 2.000 g = 30 g. of protein
Other foods: 400 g = 5 g. of protein
====
35 g.

Grains or Potatoes?

I showed you that a tribe was living in perfect health eating a diet of 90% potatoes. People who criticize potatoes are mistaken.

However, we've found a population in perfect health living on a diet of 90% grains or bread. On the other hand, many poor populations in Africa or during the middle ages ate a lot of bread and suffered from tuberculosis, arthritis, excess mucus, kidney stones, influenza, bronchitis, frequent colds, diabetes, etc.

The Hunzas, who were one of the longest-living population ever discovered, only consumed 10% grains.

The tribe found in New Guinea consumed a diet that contained on average 20 grams of protein. Most people in the Western world consume a diet that contains between 60 and 120 grams of protein, which is three times the amount consumed by the tribe. That's why the Standard American Diet—or SAD diet— makes everybody sick.

The amount of fat consumed in the New Guinea tribe's diet, when all foods are taken into account, is between 4 and 6 grams a day. This is the equivalent of a small teaspoon of oil. When we see the quantities of butter and oil that people gobble down every day, we also understand why their arteries are blocked.

Sweet potatoes and fruits and vegetables naturally contain a small percentage of fat. Adding any type of fat, such as butter or oil, is completely unnecessary. Even avocados contain too much fat and should be limited.

What struck me in this report by Dr. Bircher was the sentence "In spite of this spartan diet... the tribe was in perfect health." They should have written: "Thanks to this spartan diet..."

Half Cooking and Raw Meat

Strong-Tasting Vegetables

During the evening chats I organize every day of the year for people fasting at my center, I often get the comment that it's possible to eat every vegetable raw, such as cabbage, cauliflower, turnips, Brussels sprouts, young artichokes, etc.

I always respond:

Perfect. If you can eat all these vegetables raw, in sufficient quantities, then there's no need for cooking them. Eat them raw...but wait, make sure that you're not just trying to sustain yourself on a tiny portion just to say that you could eat them raw, like a little piece of cauliflower. You should be able to eat 200 or 300 grams, if not a pound, without cheating! That means without adding strong seasonings to hide their taste, such as vinegar, salt, and herbs.

Personally, I find all these vegetables (and many others) too strong for my delicate palate. I find it impossible to eat them raw. If I should only limit myself to the few vegetables that I can enjoy eating raw, then there wouldn't be much left in my diet!

That's why I cook these vegetables, but never the ones that pass the test of the taste buds. I merely cook them a few minutes (depending on the size and toughness) to eliminate any strong, astringent, or spicy taste.

Onions, beet leaves, leeks, potatoes, and many other vegetables cannot be eaten raw. But cooking them will make them enjoyable to eat. Onions will only need a few minutes, beets leaves 10 minutes, and leeks will cook for 20 to 30 minutes.

Jerusalem artichokes are excellent raw or cooked.

I also cook those tough cauliflower leaves, and I peel and slice the stems before cooking them, as well, at the bottom of the pot. Tough cabbage leaves will need more cooking and should be cut in smaller pieces.

Raw onion and garlic are very damaging to the kidneys and can cause inflammation, and sometimes blood in the urine and stools. I knew lady—a Romanian dentist, who put raw garlic all over her food, which caused her to see blood in her urine. Apart from this, this lady followed a hygienic diet pretty strictly.

The variety of vegetables that can be enjoyed raw is too limited to satisfy our need for variety. Already, the hygienic diet is too monotonous, compared to traditional foods.

A Varied Diet

In most families, the person in charge of the household makes sure that meals are varied from day to day. The same type of food is not served again before 15 days, on average. For example, we may eat pasta one day, or rice the next, or fish the third day, and chicken the fourth, and so on. The variety of foods is sure to appeal to all taste buds.

We've gotten in the habit since childhood of varying our meals. But gorillas don't do that. They eat the same thing all the time. Who can go back to this rather natural simplicity?

Many people get a good amount of their pleasure from the food they eat. How can we not feel frustrated to see the same foods in our plates day after day? Our civilized mind can no longer feel satisfied with simplicity. Elaborate, gourmet meals can bring us a lot of pleasure, but our health will suffer as a consequence.

That's why I tried varying the evening meal as much as I could. One night, I suggest serving cooked vegetables, and potatoes with raw greens the next day. It's best to only eat three kinds of cooked vegetables at a time, and save others for the next meal.

I therefore tolerate cooking, but only for vegetables that can't be eaten raw. Those who are happy eating everything raw don't have to cook anything. They don't even have to own a cooking pot!

I should point out again, that you should be able to eat raw vegetables in sufficient quantities without hiding their taste with salt and vinegar. Those condiments cannot be part of a hygienic diet (but lemon juice and some olive oil can be tolerated).

If you eat ridiculous quantities of vegetables you're eventually going to feel frustrated and eventually compensate by eating bread and or another unhealthy foods. Then, you'll complain about cravings...

Who can eat leeks and beets raw? It's not easy. And why should you deprive yourself of such delicious, healthy foods when a bit of cooking can render them delicious, and enjoy more variety in your diet?

List of Vegetables That Can Be Enjoyed Raw

- Cucumbers
- Winter squash
- Endives
- Fennel
- Carrots
- Celery
- Celeriac
- Peeled zucchini (the skin is bitter)
- Oyster plant
- Jerusalem artichokes
- Red, green or yellow peppers
- Peas

List of Vegetables That Can Be Cooked

- Red, white and green cabbage
- Cauliflower
- Brussels sprouts
- Artichokes
- Green beans
- Potatoes
- Cauliflower stems
- Summer squash
- Beets
- Leeks
- Garlic
- Onion
- Turnips
- Rutabagas

- Celery leaves
- Parsnips
- Sweet potatoes

How to Get in the Habit of Eating Raw Vegetables

According to Dr. Herbert N. Shelton, to get in the habit of eating raw vegetables, we should try eating a little bit every day before our meals, when we're hungry, gradually increasing quantities every day. According to his theory, we'll eventually enjoy every vegetable raw. It's a question of habit.

There's no problem when it comes to carrots, fennel, cucumber, and bell peppers. But when we first try those tough green beans, a few people may find them hard to swallow. Eventually, taste buds can adapt.

Raw Meat and Fish

The fact that raw foods have many health benefits is not a good enough reason to eat raw meat and fish. In France, we saw the rise of a movement called *Instinctive Eating*, which advocated a 100% raw food diet, including meat and fish.

Guy-Claude Burger, the instigator of this health philosophy, tried to reproduce the diet of prehistoric humans. Going back in history, we know that before the mastery of fire, humans ate everything raw.

We know that primitive men, living under the hot sun of the tropics, lived on a diet of delicious fruits as found in nature. However, a small part of the human race, lost in Europe, where the climate was hostile and cold during the winter, was forced to hunt in order to survive. This cave man is now extinct.

Another tiny part of the human race—the Eskimos—was lost in the Arctic and survived eating raw fish.

In modern days, followers of *Instinctive Eating* tried to imitate the diet of primitive men, but only followed the worst example—that of the cave men or Eskimos.

Only a part of the human race lived mainly on a diet of meat and fish. But most of ancient humans lived in the tropics, largely on a fruit-based diet.

It's also important to follow the diet that we are physiologically designed to eat—and NOT to go back to our ancestral diet. A study of comparative anatomy and physiology shows us clearly what diet we are designed to eat.

A natural hygienist doesn't eat meat or fish—whether raw or cooked—except in rare occasions for those who can't stick to their diet and occasionally cheat.

Deficiencies

A deficiency means that something is lacking. A disease caused by deficiency is a disease, "caused by the absence of essential constituents in the diet."

The main deficiency diseases are: scurvy, pellagra, osteomalacia, and anemia. Many more other diseases are partly or entirely attributed to deficiencies. Many other diseases are also attributed—entirely or partially—to deficiencies.

The largest part of our knowledge on deficiency diseases is based on animal experimentation. In these experiments, a deficiency is deliberately created. The results of these experiments are often considered definitive. In other words, researchers surmise that since a deficiency disease can be caused by a deficient diet, deficiency diseases are the result of dietary deficiencies. But this is rarely the case, as I will demonstrate next.

Deficiencies Come From Poor Assimilation

" My point of view is the opposite of what is generally accepted. Deficiency diseases are rarely caused by deficient diets, but come, in most cases, from a faulty metabolism. It means that we do not benefit from what we eat. For example, we may not be able to assimilate calcium, even though the diet may be abundant in it.

"I do not deny, however, the existence of famines or extreme situations—on a boat, in prison, or caught in a wreck in the middle of the ocean. I do not ignore the possibility of malnutrition. In Africa, famine is rampant and the deaths are in the hundreds of thousands each year, among them children, adults, and even animals. I do not deny also the damages of the denatured diets that are nearly universal."
— Herbert Shelton

Anemia

In the case of anemia, there is an iron deficiency in the subject, since the analysis shows it. But when we scrutinize the patient's menu, we notice that in most cases there plenty of iron in the diet. In fact, in pernicious anemia there is an excess of iron-based pigments in all the internal organs. The researcher J. Hunter even discovered that in fatal cases, large amounts of iron taken from the circulation could be found in the spleen. This shows that there is more than enough iron than what is needed in the bodies of anemic people.

Another proof that anemia is not caused by a lack of iron in the diet is that this disease slowly disappears during fasting, at a time when no food is eaten, and no iron is provided to the body through the diet.

During a short fast, we notice a marked increase in the red blood cell count. This demonstrates that there are adequate iron reserves in the body, but that for some reason, these reserves are not used. This proves that the iron found in their food, and subsequently, the iron accumulated in their tissues, has not been appropriated. Assimilation is failing. This is called a faulty metabolism. In these cases, we are not witnessing an iron deficiency in the menu, but rather, a lack of iron absorption.

```
"Medicine prescribes iron in cases of anemia, but this
program fails in every case. The failure is so evident, so
persistent, and has been for so many decades, that we
wonder why this treatment has not been abandoned for a long
time. The iron provided is usually in the form of a
pharmaceutical preparation, but as we have showed it, it is
unused and even harmful."
```
— Herbert Shelton

In addition, when iron is prescribed in a food form, such as in artichoke extracts, positive results are not obtained. What then do we gain in filling up the anemic person with iron-rich foods, when he/she already possesses in their tissues abundant, yet unused iron reserves because it cannot be assimilated?

The Use of Iron Is Subject to Many Factors:

- The nutritional status of the individual and the state of his/her intestinal flora

- The state of the iron consumed, whether it be biological or mineral.

- The absence of associated dietary factors in the menu, such as iron and copper—which, in turn, leads to an iron deficiency by rebound.

- The result is that an intake of iron-rich foods is not sufficient to insure proper iron utilization by the body. Often, we do not benefit from what we eat.

- Anemia is often found in obese people. Allopathic medicine imagines an iron deficiency, but when doctors prescribe iron, they are not able to correct the deficiency. In fact, the mineral elements in a pharmaceutical form cannot correct this deficiency.

  Giving these people "nourishing and solid foods" doesn't bring results either. Aren't they already obese?

- Even naturopaths, who often times follow the lead of allopathic medicine, prescribe iron-rich natural foods or artichoke extracts. The result is always poor, because these anemic people do not assimilate iron, even from a biological source. Liver and liver extracts are also useless, even though they contain an abundance of iron assimilated by the animal. And still, during a short fast we witness a rapid improvement in the blood of anemic people. We also see this in the bones of patients with rickets.

- The effect of the sun to prevent the development of rickets, in spite of a defective diet also shows, without the shadow of a doubt, that in the majority of deficiency cases, factors outside of the diet are the main cause.

We see that in anemia it is not sufficient to provide iron, but rather, it is essential that the patient be able to utilize and appropriate it. But since his or her digestive and assimilative functions may be altered, he or she will not benefit from the iron consumed, unless these functions are restored. When digestion and assimilation are faulty, for any reason, this leads to deficiencies. This applies just as well to both vitamin and mineral deficiencies.

So let's forget about chemistry for a while, and let's remember that the body takes an active part in the use of the elements that we give it.

The Intestinal Flora

The essential factor is the state of the intestinal flora. If it is in good condition, then we don't get anemia or any other deficiency disease. But if this precious flora is dying, altered, or destroyed, then the body bends under the burden of serious diseases.

What damages the intestinal flora? The damage is caused by antibiotics, drugs, alcohol, coffee, tobacco, allopathic medications taken regularly, spices, and an excess of protein rich foods. The intestinal flora is comprised by innumerable cultures of bacteria and microbes, all useful for the organic chemistry.

But how can we enrich our intestinal flora? Are you are looking for products to enrich it? Why not start by eliminating all the products that destroy it: antibiotics, drugs, chemical products (there are several, but two common examples are household cleaners and perfumes), spices, condiments, medications, alcohol, coffee, tea, etc.

With time, the flora builds itself back up with the help of foods rich in bacteria: lettuce, unwashed greens, wild plants, and other raw vegetables not mentioned.

The Natural Hygienic Diagnosis

When a patient comes to me with a deficiency determined by a laboratory analysis, I immediately try to find the causes. I analyze the habits of the subject, his family environment, his eating habits, his state of mind, the poisons he takes (or that he used to take), the stress in his life, how much sleep he is getting, etc. There is a cause for everything. Everything must be examined to find the cause for this lack of assimilation.

The patient cannot diagnose himself. He can make judgmental mistakes. For example, he could imagine that the fact that he took antibiotics for fifteen days last year may have affected the iron assimilation in his body. However, time must have eliminated the effects of these poisons. For them to be harmful in the long-term, drugs must be taken more frequently.

On the other hand, worries, sadness, and anxiety will create as many deficiencies as an unhealthy diet. Emotional irritations, frustrations, internal and family conflicts, or deceptions—these are some of the common causes of nutritional problems.

In addition to correcting these habits, sick people will require physical and mental rest. They could even need a physiological rest (a fast), but they surely don't need exams, tests, analysis, drugs, or remedies. It is only once the causes have been identified and corrected that it will be possible to restore a normal nutrition for these patients.

On top of a lifestyle change, these patients will need to physically and mentally rest. They might even need to fast (physiological rest) but there is no need for examination, tests, analyzes, drugs nor remedies.

Primary and Secondary Causes

"Deficiencies in the body do not always indicate—in fact they rarely do—a deficiency in the diet. It is a fact that it is easy to demonstrate that food intake may be more than adequate for the individual needs, but that at the same time, these needs are not being satisfied.

The nutritional deficiencies coming from a deficient diet have been qualified primary deficiencies, while those coming from a defective digestion, absorption, or utilization have been called secondary deficiencies."
—Herbert Shelton

Do We Have to Seek Calcium Rich Foods?

When the body is in a state of low alkalinity, also called acidosis, calcium, however abundant in the diet, will not be properly used. However, an increase in the alkalinity of the blood favors calcium utilization.

Where can this acidosis, which prevents calcium utilization, come from? Simply, from the excess consumption of protein foods: nuts and seeds, meat, fish, seafood, cheese, etc. In order to assimilate calcium, the first step will be to eliminate these acidifying foods.

Iron is usually abundant in the diet and body tissues of anemic people. But their body is not able to utilize it in the building of their blood. Food does not mean nutrition. Eating does not signify that we always benefit from what we eat.

Food is only the building block of nutrition. When nutrition is deficient, whatever the cause may be, the utilization of nutritional materials is paralyzed.

This shows the error of nutritional supplements—as well as the dubious search for foods rich in certain elements.

A common deficiency is vitamin D. In this case, even if many calcium-rich foods are eaten, calcium is not assimilated. This may be the case in many intestinal diseases, where assimilation can also be is faulty. Chronic indigestion alters the assimilation of iron and calcium, as well as the assimilation of many other minerals.

In many cases of physical and mental distress, vitamins and minerals consumed in sufficient quantities through the foods consumed, will nevertheless present clinically as deficiencies in the body.

It is futile to prescribe more and more vitamin and mineral supplements to such patients. Since they are incapable of absorbing and assimilating the vitamins and minerals they are already taking in, this can only further burden a nutritive system that is already impaired. The solution is to restore nutritional efficiency by improving their digestion and assimilation. These steps must be taken if the patient is to benefit from the food he eats.

When the stomach is hyper-acidic, digestion is altered. This hyper-acidity must be corrected first, before the patient can assimilate iron, calcium, etc.

Why Certain People Get Away With It?

I said that a deficient diet was not necessarily the cause of organic deficiencies. It is rare that a diet is 100% deficient. The body has the capacity to compensate for what it lacks with the help of its rich intestinal flora. In many cases, people find themselves in the same situation as those who do not take regular sunbaths, but who nonetheless benefit from the sun when occasionally exposing their hands and faces to the few rays they manage to get.

However, such a deficient diet in the long run, will end up altering the capacity of the body to assimilate correctly. Digestion, absorption, and assimilation will start degrading.

Those eat a bit of everything, such as bread, meat, lettuce, fruit, etc., but frugally, do not suffer from any deficiencies. Why? Because the damage caused by toxic foods is limited. Since cooking does not destroy the totality of vitamins, that minimal amount of raw fruits and vegetables sufficiently delays the deadline of disease. These people manage to fare better than others who constantly overeat on rich, nutritious foods.

A biological transmutation is the capacity of the body to transform one mineral into another. This remarkable discovery, made by the French researcher Louis Kervan, can explain how some diets that lack certain nutrients do not always lead to deficiencies.*

To avoid deficiencies, these steps should be implemented, as outlined. They are listed in order of priority, which must be respected in all circumstances:

1) Before eating anything, wait for genuine, true hunger.

2) It is preferable to select foods specific to humans, raw and in their natural state, without harmful seasonings or even aromatic herbs.

3) Avoid cooking as much as possible—without making a religion out of it.

* **NOTES BY FP:** Biological transmutations have not been proven scientifically. However, this doesn't significantly alter Mosséri's message and advice for better health and digestion.

And What About Organic Food?

As Shelton said "When people eat organic food in excess without being able to benefit from it, there is no point in giving them more whatever the form: food supplements, concentrates, extracts. They are not helped with mineral extracts and vitamin concentrates. The one and only way to help them is by suppressing the causes maintaining the nutritional alteration and by prescribing enough rest to allow their body to restore normal secretions and excretions."

Suppressing the cause is often sufficient to restore a normal situation. But keep in mind that a cause is often complex.

"Over nutrition of a toxemic patient, thinking he will be able to effectively use the food, that is beyond ridiculous.

"Over nutrition of a profoundly unbalanced patient and hoping for good digestion and food absorption is like planting carrots and hoping to harvest potatoes!" said Shelton.

Chemicals

Medicine does not realize that nutrition is something other than a simple chemical reaction made in a laboratory. They talk about calcium, iron, vitamins, etc., when they should be talking about natural foods.

Nature placed all its nutritional treasures in balanced quantities in the foods that we eat. We need to eat these natural foods in such a way that we derive as many benefits from them as possible.

Arshavir Ter-Hovanessian, the author of *Raw Eating*, understood this problem more than anyone else. We eat cabbage, lettuce, apples, oranges, and other organic and living foods, but not iron, phosphorus, or vitamin B. When a food contains calcium, it simultaneously contains thousands of other elements that have yet to be discovered.

Magnesium Chloride

It is quite easy to see that magnesium chloride, which is so often recommended by naturopaths, is as efficient as the useless mineral and chemical salts. This product cannot be assimilated because of its mineral—instead of vegetal—origin (it is inert and non-living).

"The so-called biochemist," said Shelton, " is not aware of the requirements of the body." And will never know about them by the way. How then could he brag about fulfilling the requirements, even if his artificial mix was usable?

The one and only way to fulfill the body nutritional needs is by providing it with specific, natural and whole foods – that have not been transformed nor altered.

Why does the body eliminate chemical salts, like magnesium chloride, so rapidly? Because they are useless, Mr. Geoffroy. Stop imitating medicine and pharmacopeia.

Trace Elements

Some elements were discovered in the human body in such small amounts that they are known as "traces," These include: copper, tin, nickel, chromium, manganese, caesium, lithium, palladium, molybdenum, rubidium, selenium, strontium, tellurium, germanium, and vanadium.

Copper and nickel have a specific and common purpose to play in the body, but it is not known if the other elements are useful, or if they are just here as foreign substances.

It is also not known how many other elements are present but impossible to detect with current methods.

Nevertheless, one thing is not a mystery anymore: it is possible to provide the body with all the rare elements it needs in the required proportions and combinations, as if they were provided by food. Natural food from Nature provides us with the elements we need in a form our body can use. Nothing else can provide us with what we really need.

Trace elements synthesized in laboratories are chemicals. But our organisms are only able to use the elements from biologic origin.

Relative Importance of Organic Foods

How important is organic food when compared to other health factors?

Organic foods are an obsession for some health food enthusiasts, but when they get sick they go straightaway to the physician and get drugs! A single pill or tablet contains as much chemicals as 100 kg of chemically treated apples.

So there is inconsistency: we try avoiding chemicals by eating organic food but on the other hand we don't hesitate in taking medication to for our symptoms. People would love that medicine could combine with naturopathy but they struggle to understand they are fundamentally different. People love the idea of "alternative medicine" but do not really accept the fact this kind of medicine does not suppress the symptoms.

People know drugs are harmful but believe it is mandatory to use them.

Food grown with chemicals contains infinitesimal toxic poisons traces. Eating commercial foods is insignificant when compared to taking prescription drugs. If the aim is to suppress chemical products, then the first step should be to stop using prescription drugs.

If you buy chemically grown fruits, peal them before eating them. For lettuce, throw away the first two rows of leaves that would be wilted anyway. Wash the leaves with water.

Conclusion

To overcome deficiencies, we must eliminate the causes: drugs, spices, coffee, wine, tea, etc. Then, we must eat a diet of water-rich foods, specifically, raw fruits and vegetables, and very small quantities of foods that are high in protein. A water fast detoxifies the body and automatically improves the assimilation of the necessary elements. Do not fast more than your health and reserves allow you to. `(Please see a competent hygienic practitioner if and when planning a fast—FP)` I do not recommend doing blood tests after such a fast, but if you insist, please wait several months before doing them.

There Are Four Things To Do

1. The first one is: to eliminate the causes.

2. The second is less important in the short term, but very important in the long term: to return to natural foods.

3. Fasting also allows detoxifying the organism and systematically improves the assimilation of the required substances. Do not fast more than your health allows. Always fast under supervision.

4. Do not undertake blood tests after a few months after the end of such a cure.

Is One Man's Food Another Man's Poison?

We often think that what is appropriate for one person could not be ideal for another. We even say that what is food for someone can be poison for someone else. Is this true?

We don't say that cows are so different from each other that they must be fed differently. We don't say that sheep are so different from one another that different foods must be given to each of them. Why then should human beings be so different from each other, to the point where we must give meat to some, and grains to others?

There is an old saying that states, "One man's food is another man's poison." Based on this, many people are opposed to a uniform diet for everyone, because they say that what could be good for some may be harmful to others.

The Answer from Natural Hygienists

Hygienists will reply to this by saying that, "The study of anatomy and physiology proves that every living organism, a man or a woman being no exception, possesses an innate relationship with the food that provides it the best material for its nutrition."

In other words, nature provides a specific food for every species according to its anatomy and physiology, so that it may be able to use it in the most efficient way to fill its nutritional needs.
Hygienists also stated that the human species is subjected to the same natural laws that govern all other species regarding the specific foods appropriated to it by nature.

"Man's body is constituted according to a very precise model. The principles that rule the constitution of man, through which he grows, develops himself, expresses his strength, and maintains his structures and actions, keeps the integrity of his structures and of his life—these principles are applicable to every human being."

"One man alone, in its organic principles of its constitution and in the sphere of action of the main fundamental laws through which his life is determined—one man alone is the archetype of the race."

"The special differences, which are, in fact, very small, and mainly pathological, are subjected to the greater uniformity. These divergences do not change in anyway the great constituents that belong to all. Essentially and in all its elements of excellence—physical, mental, and moral—all men are the same."
—Herbert Shelton

(Please note: The word "man" is a generic term that comprises both men and women.—A.M.)

As far as life is concerned, the Laws of Nature are the same for every human being. This is not a law that applies only in certain circumstances—it is an immutable, universal fact.

Generally speaking, what maintains life in one man, will also maintain life in another, and what kills one man, will kill another man.

Appropriate For One, But Not Appropriate For Another?

"If it were true that one's food could not be appropriate to another, what would happen with our eating in society? We would constantly be brought to be on our guards and avoid poisons! It would be of no help to know that others have eaten a certain food without problems — since what is good for them could poison us. And how, furthermore, could we judge others? By preparing a menu for others, whose needs are completely foreign to us, how could we avoid poisoning them? Would we ask to each guest that agrees to eat with us that he prepare us, in advance, a list of the foods that he can eat without danger?"

"How would we establish the menus in schools, hospitals, prisons, etc., if the old saying were true? And the restaurants and hotels, how would they prepare the menus?"

"If the old saying were true, how would farmers know what foods to grow? And how would merchants know what they must buy for selling to the public?"

"If this saying were true, the market and industry would be in a state of complete confusion. Even mothers wouldn't know if, after nursing their babies, if their milk is a food or a poison for them."

"Are we giving too much attention to this old saying? Certainly, but where stops its application, if there is one? But we understand it as the expression of a confused state into which humanity got lost with its habits, when it contains bitter sarcasm."

"The fact is that the saying is never utilized with consistency, nor intelligence. It is used only by the person who has no reply to give, when we urge him to consider the importance of healthy eating habits."
—Herbert Shelton

Would it be a physiological benefit for some to go to bed early, while others of a different constitution are able to stay up late at night without any problems?

It is obvious that sleep is indispensable to all, but the needs for each person may be different. Certain people need to sleep ten hours a night, while others can get by with only five or six. This does not in any way contradict the rule that sleep is necessary to all.

The same can be said for food. Is it possible that some may be well adapted to eating frugally, while others are better adapted to a gluttonous diet? Some people may need to eat more than others when using hunger as their guideline.

Personal Intolerances

The human race as a whole has the same constitution. However, variations can exist from person to person, but these are just pathological deviations from the norm. These variations can only justify certain accommodations here and there, depending on the human being.

On the other hand, personal intolerances are all shortcomings specifically tied to an individual, but they do not discredit the fundamental diet specifically meant for the whole human race.

For example, there are certain individuals whose system cannot adequately handle large quantities of acid fruits (strawberries, citrus, etc.), since they themselves may be acidified as a result of an unhealthy diet. After a change in their dietary practices, they will be able to eat more acid fruit without experiencing much, if any, discomfort. But until a new diet is implemented, these foods will have to be avoided.

There are some people who cannot tolerate raw vegetables because their intestines have been weakened by prescription drugs. In these cases, they will have to be introduced them little by little, starting with vegetable juices.

There are other personal intolerances or specific individual adaptations that justify changes in the diet. This does not change the basis of the diet, or the fact that every human being, in ideal conditions, will thrive on the same foods and influences.

Grains Are Not Our Natural Food

The True Natural Hygienist

All true Hygienists are opposed to grains. This include bread, pasta, rice, flour, cookies, crackers, etc.

It seems very difficult for most people to understand this subject, because unconsciously they refuse to abandon the habit of eating bread and other grain products.

Those who call themselves Hygienists and still promote bread, even whole wheat, are not true Hygienists. They don't understand that Nature doesn't produce bread, that grains are meant to be eaten by birds, who are granivores (a granivore is a grass eater, a granivore is a grain eater), and that humans are frugivores (also eaters of fruits and some green leaves).

There are many reasons why grains are not suited for humans. Among the most valid ones are those taken from the science of biology—the same type of arguments that vegetarians use to condemn meat eating.

A chart of comparative anatomy reveals that humans have none of the characteristics of the carnivore. They do not have appropriate teeth to bite the prey, nor an adequate liver to neutralize all the toxins, and so on. Everybody can understand this easily; humans are not carnivores.

But what I say is that humans are not granivores either. We are not biologically designed to eat grains. For every class of animals on the planet, Nature has provided a certain category of foods for them. Any deviation from that will create all sorts of problems: disease, cancer, etc.

A machine that is supposed to function well with a certain type of oil will not function as well with a different type of oil. It will clog up and break down. This is the major argument against grains. All other "scientific" arguments are only about details.

Nature has provided a special type of food for fish, another type of food for cows, and something entirely different for bears. And for us, Nature provides us with our natural food: fruits and vegetables.

Nature is not a chaos. Every species eats the food they were designed to eat. If horses would start eating meat, and lions start grazing with the cows, it would be the end of everything.

Bread and grains, even whole grains, are extremely deficient in minerals, compared to fruits and greens. Grains are lacking in alkaline minerals like calcium. They are indeed some of the most acid-forming foods. Our physiology is not designed to handle the digestion of grains.

The ptyalin enzyme in our mouth can only handle a small amount of starch found in roots and some fruits. Species that are like some types of birds, have a special stomach called the gizzard. What is a gizzard?

It's a sort of second stomach that permits certain types of bird to grind hard seeds in order to digest them. With that type of strong stomach, they can even pulverize little rocks in no time. In fact, they swallow rocks to help grind grains. Even needles, swallowed by some young birds, are broken into pieces, and eliminated with no apparent damage.

Have you ever seen chickens and other types of fowl eat rocks, nails, and other hard and indigestible things? At that moment, you probably asked yourself: why are these animals eating these useless and harmful things? Have they gone mad? Or are they simply following to their instinct? They are simply introducing hard things into their gizzard to help grind the hard seeds that they just ate.

Birds and fowl have no teeth. That's why they have to swallow whole seeds. But since they need to digest them, Nature provides them with a most perfect grinding machine, attached to their stomach. Small rocks, when eaten, are used as millstones.

But humans are much different. They do not have a gizzard. They cannot grind hard seeds like grains or legumes. That is why those foods are not meant for us.

Now someone will say that we can replace the gizzard with a millstone, constructed by humans, and cook the grains, to soften them and render them easy to chew and digest; and that's about what we've been doing for several thousands of years. But this does not solve the problem.

The digestive tract of humans, of all frugivores, is too long for an adequate digestion of heavy starches. These foods stay there for too long, and thus have a tendency to ferment. Grains are natural foods for birds and fowl, but not humans, who are not equipped with a gizzard and other physiological designs, in order to process grain properly.

Furthermore, humans cannot eat and enjoy these foods in their natural state. They are simply not foods we are biologically meant to eat. Our natural foods are fruits, roots, vegetables and green leaves.

When Medicine Condemns a Sick Person

Once in a while, it happens that a doctor, brought to a sick person's bedside, condemns him to death, in the short or long term.

"He only has a few months or a few years to live," she will say to loved ones with a solemn and grave look, with a distressed pity or a faked compassion, as appropriate for the occasion. But is she Almighty God, to affirm with so much certitude, so much authority, an approaching end?

Of course, after years of beating up a sick organism, intoxicating it with chemical products, suppressing symptoms, treating this then that, loading it with foods it cannot digest, and considering the very skim reserves that it still possessed—doctors can predict, with some accuracy, its forthcoming end.

But does not medicine itself contribute to create this degeneration, this end, with a morbid precision that recalls chemical weaponry?

In effect, medicine can predict death coming in two years, exactly like the military can launch a rocket and reach a target, located five thousand miles away, with a margin of error of 30 feet. Both are rarely wrong, because when it comes to death, medicine and the military are careful programmers.

Starting from their dismal prognosis, sensitive souls prefer to shorten the suffering of the sick, bringing their instantaneous death by euthanasia.

Yet tribunals show clemency in front of a moved public—unsuspecting of certain abuses— and the guilty and criminals are released with a light sentence.

Let's be frank: it is an unspeakable crime to want to kill a sick person when medicine condemns him. How many times did medicine err in its prognosis? Often. Very often.

Claude was also condemned

Claude is a Belgian who suffered from liver cirrhosis. Medicine gave him 3-5 years to live. I consulted Shelton's book, the 7th volume of Hygienic System, to find that his prognosis is the same, probably copied from Dr. J.H. Tilden's book. The cause was alcohol, replaced by abuse of sugar, of which he consumed one or two handfuls a day.

The man fasted for 40 days at my place, and returned home satisfied, because the daily depressions that used to accompany his drinking were gone. Ten years later, an athlete with an impressive set of muscles came to visit me. It was he—Claude! He was not dead, but actually living and enjoying radiant health.

If he had followed the classical medical treatment, he probably would not have lived over 5 years. Thus, the medical prognosis only concerns those that follow the medical road. It cannot be confirmed when the patient changes course, as did Claude.

So many desperately sick people, feeling that the drugs were making them suffer more than their own disease, and "knowing" that death will be meeting them anyhow, abandon all medical treatments. So many of them prefer to die without getting the help of anyone, and without being rushed. If they have to die anyway, why take useless pharmaceutical chemical products?

That's when the miracle happens. To the great surprise of everybody, and in spite of their doctors, these dying people, abandoned at the threshold of their graves, who threw away all hope and drugs, do not die! They live, in spite of all doomsaying, in a crushing refutation of the pathetic medical prognosis.

And those that wanted to send them to Heaven, by pity, through euthanasia? Are they not committing an unspeakable crime? They believe in medicine like others believe in the Dear Lord.

Thus, stopping the medical treatment sufficed to extend the lives of these seriously sick persons, and sometimes to recover totally, especially when they changed methods.

Natural Hygiene, and to a lesser degree the other natural methods that are less scientific, have contributed to the cure of thousands of incurables condemned by medicine.

When doctors condemn a sick person, their prognosis will only end up being right if the patient continues with treatment.

Again, medicine cannot predict what will happen to a seriously sick person who does not treat himself. They never observed such a case, nor studied its physiological behaviors. It could not interest them, because it would signify their own uselessness.

Valérie's True Story

In the 80's, television made a lot of noise about little Valérie. Affected with leukemia, she was subjected to the barbaric treatment of cortisone and other pharmaceutical poisons. To what end, since medicine had condemned her? To relieve her, alleviate her pains, and delay the fatal date—so they said. It was quite easy to affirm it without proofs, because medicine does not have proofs for what it affirms, only for abridged statistics. [Any honest statistician will admit that statistics can only indicate a correlation of factors, not a causal connection between them. -F.P.]

But why not affirm, with as much confidence, if not more, that this treatment increased her pain, and dragged her faster to her end?

The journalists interviewed the girl's doctor, Professor Olive, then Valérie, and finally her mother. Generally, journalists are on the medical side. But this scandal seemed profitable enough for them to betray medicine, especially since public opinion had been changing for some time in favor natural medicines.

The hormone treatment forced on Valerie, who was nine years old at the time, led to awful pains instead of their alleviation. Since she was injected with male hormones, hair grew all over her body and face. She had to shave and even burn these hairs.

The treatment finished— without positive results, of course, but negative ones, as we have just seen—and the doctors wanted to start this criminal treatment all over again. What results did they expect? They could not say. Was it just an experiment to them?

The little girl, facing even more of the callous and bumptious treatment, refused at once. They were handling her body, and she intended to remain in control of it, in defiance of medicine who wanted to appropriate it. Besides which, a serious symptom also started to manifest itself—capillaries started to burst out all over her small, bruised body.

On television, the journalists, well aware of the magnitude of their betrayal—they who are usually so servile to medicine—declared right at the beginning that their documentary should not be taken as an attack against the Faculty. It was however, but their warning glossed it over. They schemed to attenuate the blows, to profit from the scandal, and at the same time, hold back the waves of antipathy that it could engender.

Valérie declared that all the medical treatments she received were only experiments on her body, done without her initial agreement, and that she preferred to die at home. She went back home, and they could not prevent it. At least, not at the moment.

They had told her that the treatment gave 70% of positive results, but she quickly replied,

"They showed me no proofs for that."

The accuracy and maturity of her words showed that there was someone behind her—a dissident practitioner who was telling her what to say and what to answer. In fact, we learned afterward that her mother had consulted an homeopath.

Professor Olive, (her real name), was upset that her prey was going back home, slamming the hospital door behind her.

Was it a hospital or a prison? More a prison, but without bars. The sick are not easily released. They are held by all manner of intimidation, pressure, threats and laws.

Seeing the needless sufferings of her daughter, the mother sought without success to meet with Professor Olive. Impossible to see her, not even for a minute. It's the same everywhere with these doctors and directors of hospitals. We can never meet them. They flee, they hide.

And the nurses? They have one rule, the same everywhere: Say nothing to patients or parents, so that nothing can be used against the staff in case of accident. Let slip only soothing, evasive words—quickly, on the go, like a thief who does not want to be seen.

Everywhere and in every hospital, it's the same.

So Valérie came back home and called a homeopath. Surely that's what explained, her phrases, full of maturity. For a balanced, thoughtful, nine year-old girl, someone else had to stand behind her to whisper the right words.

But Professor Olive—not a green olive, but a real black one—did not consider the game lost. She held on to her prey, like the eagle to the sparrow. She lodged a complaint with the Children's Court. A hearing occurred and the tribunal ordered the mother to send Valérie back to the hospital.

But, since when do judges settle scientific problems and controversies?

Especially when Professor Olive had against her a registered homeopathic physician, who, like her, had studied medicine and was fully accredited. Or else, allopathic medicine becomes the state medicine, just like Catholic religion was once the state religion. Having abolished state religion, it is time to abolish state medicine and leave the citizens free to practice the religion and medicine they prefer.

"So," exclaimed Valérie on television, in front of millions of astounded viewers, "we cannot die where we want? We cannot die at home?" But her mother was determined not to give up. Probably supported by the homeopath, she went on appeal. She won, and the girl stayed home, no longer fearing the leaders of the Faculty, which had become oppressive and dictatorial. But it was not over!

The little Valérie, who was condemned by medicine, did not die, according to their miserable prognosis. Of course, this prognosis was based on continuation of the treatment, and could no longer apply as soon as this treatment was discontinued.

Her condition improved so much that she was able to go back to school and resume her interrupted studies.

So many sick people, after having tried all the official medicines and physicians, one after the other, finally see an "outlaw" practitioner. At this state, these desperados are in such ruin that we can qualify them as eleventh-hour patients.

If the non-medical methods have so much success, we can only imagine the phenomenal success they would have if the sick could, at the beginning of their problems, embrace natural medicine.

Valérie is now in her twenties. She is happy and her health is better than ever. And leukemia? Only a bad memory that, nonetheless, gets the credit for opening her eyes to the inanity of medicine. And to think that some would have advocated her euthanasia because of a stupid-as-usual medical prognosis.

Wrong Physiological Norms

Medicine established certain physiological norms, but most of them are wrong.

The average "normal" pulse has been established at a pulse of 72 per minute, but physiologist simply got this number by looking at the average, from a sampling of people selected randomly. It was not considered that most people are chronically sick, and therefore their pulse is abnormally high.

Healthy people don't die at half of their life expectancy, at 70 years old instead of the 120 years our body is really capable of living. Healthy people don't get sick with an occasional cold. Healthy people don't suffer from numerous little pains and aches. In all honesty, how can we take this sick population as an average? To simply get an idea of the poor health of the population, we can just start counting the number of hospitals, drugs sold, and practicing physicians.

We know that the average pulse of athletes and very strong people is around 50 beats per minutes.

That is why, when we want to study comparative anatomy in various animals, let's not stumble upon one of the biggest obstacles there is: the average norms adopted by medicine, and by everybody. They are false!

A normal pulse should be what it would be normally, just like blood pressure, breathing, white blood cell count, body temperature, etc.

To understand the meaning of the word normal, we should acknowledge that the failed health of sick people is abnormal. The normal state of the human being is that of radiant health.

Can We Compare Ourselves to Others?

What do we see around us? We see that everyone overeats protein-rich foods: meat, fish, cheese, legumes, seafood, and eggs. In richer countries, meat is eaten in excess, while in under-developed countries (like in India or Egypt), legumes are.

So can we compare our health to the health of others, saying, "My neighbor eats meat and is healthy? My cousin drinks coffee, wine, eats cheese, enjoys his food and is doing fine?"

Beware: most people are all chronically sick, even if they appear cheerful, and even if they are happy and radiant. They don't talk about their daily misery and pains. Fatigue is fought with coffee, insomnia with sleeping pills, constipation with laxatives, pessimism with wine, depression with drugs, and headaches with aspirin. We think that they are doing well just by looking at them, but it's not true.

And those who suffer from nothing, for how long is their strong and resistant organism going to hold up? How long is it going to take before the integrity of the organs, inherited from sturdy parents, is affected by the abuse of protein-rich foods?

It's only a question of time. The fortunate people who have strong genetics will take more time to damage and degrade their bodies than those who have inherited a fragile constitution.

Of Equal Things Only...

Once again, can we compare ourselves to others in the health field? We can obviously do it, in theory, when everything is equal. But, I say in theory, because things are never equal, except maybe for twins.

The physical values of every individual, its parameters, are never identical to those of others—constitutions are different, the organs inherited do not have the same resistance, the eating habits are not the same.

Even for brothers, though from the same mother, the health, the diet, and the psychology of the mother during pregnancy was not necessarily uniform for both. When she was bearing one, she could have smoked, taken aspirins or experienced an emotional shock; when bearing the other, she could have been on vacation, relaxed and not taking any drugs or poisons.

Individuals do not have the same habits. One smokes two packs of cigarettes a day, a second drinks coffee, a third drinks wine, while a fourth eats carefully and frugally. We should never say that so-and-so smokes, drinks wine and coffee and is doing better than I, who is careful about his food and never takes any poison. Also, one can drink one cup of coffee or five. There is not the same effect on health.

Finally, there is the element of genetics that comes into play.

We Can Only Compare Ourselves To Ourselves

If we cannot compare ourselves to our neighbor or even our brother, we can very well compare ourselves to ourselves, from a period of time to another, analyzing the important factors that may have influenced our health, toward improvement or ruin.

For example, when we change diet; when we get a new job; when we are relaxed or irritable; when we take our time or simply rush to work; when we are distressed or serene; when we smoke or drink wine—all these factors influence health. We can see that very clearly. Staying up late at night or going to bed early: the result of each is not the same on our state of health.

We must also be able to distinguish the important causes from the trivial ones, which cannot be done by the neophyte without the help of an experienced and practiced natural hygienist. My views, derived from a lifetime of practical observations of myself and thousands of clients, indicate that health is a rich subject. Understanding it is a deep process, beyond the scope of casual comparisons.

The Background of Natural Hygiene and the Difference from Other Sciences

Natural Hygiene was discovered at the start of the 19th century by about twenty researchers, most of whom were medical doctors. These included the doctors: J.H. Tilden, R.T. Trall, Alcott, Jennings, Edmond Morals, Sylvester Graham, Dewey, Walter, Weger, and many others.

Many of these researchers had studied medicine, because they were themselves sick. They hoped to find in their studies the solution to their health problems. But as soon as their studies were over, they gave up medicine because they hadn't found anything in it that was useful to their health, nor for their illness.

They all had an incisive and Cartesian mind, like all good researchers. They first searched to find in medicine some basic principles, but failed to find them. They each worked on their own, alone and isolated from each other. Each one through their work, their own observations, and reasoning discovered a different aspect of natural health. They also made some mistakes along the way.

Dr. Shelton was the one who synthesized all of these sensational discoveries, having weeded out the possible mistakes, and brought everything together into a cohesive system that he called Natural Hygiene.

Thus, Natural Hygiene was discovered and developed in the United States, before spreading after to several Western countries. In France, I introduced the Hygienic System in 1950 and at the moment I'm the only one who practices it in its original pure state, without including any useless naturopathic modalities. I spread Natural Hygiene through my many books and my fasting center.

Right after the discovery of Natural Hygiene in the United States, at the end of the 19th century, Naturopathy took hold in Europe with its pioneers such as Louis Kuhne, Adolph Just, Kneipp, Priestnitz, Blitz, etc.

The Difference Between Natural Hygiene and Naturopathy

It's important to distinguish Natural Hygiene and Naturopathy. What Naturopathy tries to do is reform medicine —that Naturopathy finds too violent, too chemical and artificial—with an alternative medicine that doesn't deny the fundamental basis of traditional medicine, which is to fight disease and its symptoms.

Naturopathy uses natural methods such as:

- Hydrotherapy
- Clay
- Chiropractics
- Massages
- Herbal remedies
- Nutritional supplements
- Bioanalysis
- Acupuncture
- Homeopathy

On the other hand, Natural Hygiene does not recognize the existence of remedies—even natural ones. We state that the only "remedy," so to speak, is the elimination of the cause and not that of the symptoms, even through natural means.

When the effect is suppressed, it always comes back in one form or another. But when the cause is eliminated, the effect (the disease) is eliminated with rest and restored vitality.

Natural Hygienists only use hygienic factors necessary to life and health, and avoid everything else. For example, massages are not necessary to life and health; therefore, they should be discarded as a Hygienic factor for sick people

```
(Note by FP: What Mosséri is trying to explain here is a
key element of Natural Hygiene. He's not per se against
massages for relaxation, but simply stating the obvious,
that because massages are not essential to maintain health,
that they are not necessary to restore it as well. Human
```

touch is certainly an important factor of health, but therapeutic massages are not a health requirement. When someone is sick, they should look for the normal requirements of life and pay attention to those, and avoid the therapeutic remedies that basically only work on masking the symptoms and delaying their appearance.)

Natural Hygiene is not therapeutic. It is not a new therapy. It only seeks to eliminate the causes of diseases, which are the conditions of an unhealthy life (especially our artificial diet).

While Naturopathy tries to reform medicine, Natural Hygiene rejects it entirely in its principles and practices.

Anatomy and Physiology Are Not Medicine

Let's be careful. The study of anatomy, physiology and biology, as they are taught during the first years of medical studies, do not constitute the study of medicine per se. These sciences are perfectly valid and necessary. Modern medicine includes therapeutics—that is the treatment of diseases with drugs, as well as other injurious practices.

- "You've rejected medicine", I told my friend, Dr. J.M.C.
- "I did not disown medicine", he told me. "I only rejected drugs".
- "But medicine is drugs. Without drugs, there is no medicine anymore"

As for surgery, we certainly allow it for accidents as well as some rare irreversible cases.

Natural Hygiene is therefore a revolutionary science.

Disease and Natural Hygiene

Toxemia

Toxemia is the presence of any substance incompatible with health in the blood, lymph, fluids, organs, tissues, and cells of the body. This is what we vaguely call the *terrain*.

Dr. P. Delore writes:

```
"The notion of terrain is justified with this banal
observation, that in front of the external agent of
disease, living beings act differently. This is the cancer-
prone terrain, and not the cancerous terrain. This
distinction is essential if we want to avoid total
confusion when we talk about the terrain."
```

This naturopathic doctor that I just quoted still has a notion of disease as being a separate entity, because he talks of it coming from the "exterior." He's still swimming in the muddy oceans of medicine.

On the other hand, what he's talking about are the heredity or the individual predispositions, which he's grouping under the name "terrain." So for him, microbes will always cause disease, which will take form according to what heredity predisposes. He can then explain the diversity of diseases in individuals.

But he's completely ignoring the Hygienic concept of toxemia, according to which the terrain of each person can vary from one period to the next, from one month to the next, one day to the next, according to what one eats, what one drinks, and the poisons one takes.

But for this doctor, only microbes matter—the "external agent," as he calls it—along with the hereditary terrain. The quality of tissues and of the blood is constant in his mind. Tobacco, alcohol, coffee, and chemicals wouldn't compromise the organism. We can clearly see the deficiency in his positions.

When a person drinks alcohol, this poison can be detected immediately in the blood, and disappears after a little while, once the kidneys have filtered it out. The terrain changes according to what we drink.

When a person eats products filled with chemicals, such as canned foods and other foods made in a factory, the blood and tissues will soak up these toxins. The terrain is intoxicated. After, the body tries to eliminate these toxic products with a violent toxemia crisis.

What Is a Disease?

Disease is a compensatory process that the body initiates when the level of toxemia has gone over the tolerance level.

A disease is not an entity, something to be chased, destroyed or healed as claimed by backward modern medicine. A disease is due to a reaction of the organism, a vital process. That is not an enemy fighting the organism but an effort of elimination.

Disease is actually not a substance to fight against through chemical or natural means. This is a vital action of the organism and it is important to cooperate with it.

It is said that disease takes its course. Why do we have to take poisons then? Let it takes its course.

Natural Hygiene does not look for new remedies, therapies or sensational cures. A Natural Hygiene practitioner will never recommend any remedy, even a natural one.

Those prescribing chemical remedies are physicians. Those prescribing natural remedies are naturopaths. They are not natural hygienists, even if they claim to be in order to attract more customers who are unable to make the difference.

At first, the body can handle various poisons and unhealthy foods, but thereafter, it is saturated with them and reaches the tolerance level. It then tries to eliminate these poisons. But because the normal elimination channels are quickly overloaded, it requests other channels to help itself. This is why disease is a compensatory process.

On the other hand, disease is a toxemia crisis—an effort of violent or passive elimination—whether the disease is acute (fever, acute pains, vomiting, diarrhea) or feeble (when disease is chronic).

Disease is a vicarious elimination. Here the word "vicarious" means "compensatory." The organs of elimination being surcharged, the body requests other organs to take over and continue elimination.

In this manner, fever often helps the entire body when it is overloaded, and the normal organs of elimination (liver, kidneys, and lungs) are not able to purify it. The lungs often work, through coughing, to eliminate mucus that the nasal passage is not able to eliminate. The fact that disease is elimination is proved by the increased elimination such as: dark urine, bad breath, fever, pimples, diarrhea, vomiting, fetid perspiration, pus, etc.

The purpose of disease is to purify the body, so that it can perform better.

An acute illness will only show up if the body is overloaded with impurities caused by non-hygienic habits, when the organs of elimination mentioned are saturated above-and-beyond their capacity and that their potential of vitality is high.

```
(NOTE by FP: The last wording by Mosséri "their potential
of vitality" simply means that a weak organ will not be
able to assist in the elimination as well as a relatively
strong and healthy organ. It also alludes to the fact that
the potential of the body is limited and that the more we
abuse it, the more difficult it gets to get back our
health.)
```

The Toxemia Concept

When we sit down to eat our meals every day, they can be separated in two parts. First, the food is absorbed, assimilated and appropriated by the organism. If the food contains poisons, or if during digestion certain by-products of fermentation and putrefaction are created, those can enter the blood stream and pollute it. This is what we call the exogenous toxemia (from outside).

As this process is happening, new cells are constantly replacing old cells; the old cells then must be eliminated. The blood is cleaned of its impurities by the kidneys, which must then eliminate them through the urine. The lungs also eliminate carbon dioxide, a result of the oxidation of cellular waste, through breathing. Normal elimination is thus carried out through oxidation (breathing) of wastes, or their rejection by the kidneys through urine.

But, when enervation of the organism slows down the normal elimination of bodily wastes—just like bad news can disturb an interpreter working at United Nations. It's important to understand the term "enervation" and distinguish it from "nervousness." Everything in the body works with nervous energy. This energy must stay abundant for good functioning of all organs. Everything that risks diminishing this nervous energy, such as muscular fatigue, mental fatigue, overeating, sexual excesses, poisons, unhealthy substances, bad food, and so on—will influence elimination.

```
(Note by FP: The term "enervation" has been used by Natural
Hygienists for years to explain the process that Mosséri is
describing.)
```

When elimination is thus slowed down, the level of toxemia rises. This means that the quantity of toxins that should be eliminated rise appreciably, just like a river rises when we build a dam. With this toxemia level rising and rising, the nose will take over and start eliminating some of the toxins, through mucus (cold, sinusitis, asthma, etc.). Similarly, the elevation of the water level contained by a dam causes an increase in pressure on its walls, and the dam ends up yielding at one of its most vulnerable and weak points. We have a water leak.

Fever

If we enjoy a good level of vitality (like children), the body will raise its temperature to oxidize more rapidly the accumulated wastes that threaten its well being. This is just like a chimney that's filled with coal. The temperature rises rapidly, until the fuel supply is exhausted. Then the temperature goes down on its own.

This is the true meaning of a fever. It's a process that the body starts to help elimination.

But what is it that creates enervation in the first place? Enervation is caused by unhealthy habits, un-hygienic routines, and conditions unfavorable to life, such as: overwork (physically, mentally, or sexually), strong emotions, stress, grief, worries, overeating, alcohol, coffee, chocolate and cacao, spices, fermented cheeses, and the acidifying by-products of foods that are not biologically adapted to the human race.

(Note by FP: In the last sentence, Mosséri is referring principally to the consumption of grain, meat, beans, etc. The foods we are biologically adapted to are fruits, roots and green vegetables.)

It is certainly possible to expose ourselves to cold, humidity, and cool drafts without catching a cold, as long as we avoid thin internal uncleanliness caused by anti-hygienic habits. Being cold is, thus, a very secondary cause to enervation and to the common cold and flu.

Internal Cleanliness

In civilized countries, we place great importance to external cleanliness and no importance to internal cleanliness. We shower every day, we clean the smallest particle of dust that sets on furniture. We use abrasive products to scrub, to make shine, and improve appearances.

But, internal cleanliness of the body is much more important to health than external cleanliness. We can certainly shower three times a day, but does it matter when we're dirty on the inside?

How can we tell if we're dirty on the inside? It's simple: you just have to smell sweat under the armpits, as we've seen. It shouldn't have any smell. The stools should also be odorless and well formed. (Note by FP: Stools don't need to be "well-formed," but they should be odorless, as Mosséri mentioned, and "clean"—which means rarely necessitating the use of toilet paper. Of course, you'll use some, to "check.") The morning breath should be pure, nice and perfumed—instead of being nauseating and bad. Taste in the mouth should be sweet, not bitter, pasty or dry.

Air and sun oxidize this odorless perspiration. As for dust, it has no consequences for health. However, if we stain our hands with chemicals, for example, when we repair a bike or a car, we should quickly wash our hands. If such products could get into the body through food, the consequences could be serious—with paralysis being the worst negative outcome.

Enervation

Let's come back to the topic of enervation.

For those who are very close to the point of toxemic overload, the slightest bout of cold weather, period of overwork, or excess will have an enervating effect that will slow down elimination and throw toxemia over the level of tolerance.

This is how a cold occurs. It's just like the Torricelli's experiment, whose barrel exploded when pressure increases. (Just review your physics course, if you've gone to college!)

If, however, the toxemia level is not very high in the organism, this temporary slowdown in elimination will not be sufficient to bring the waste level over the level of tolerance, and no cold will be "caught."

Let's clarify again that enervation doesn't mean "nervousness" or stress, which would be limited to upset nerves. Enervation is a word in physiology, which means the drainage of vital nervous energies.

The nervous system oversees all functions of the body and directs them masterfully, like a great orchestra conductor. It leads the digestive, respiratory, secretary, execratory, muscular, sexual, and eliminative functions—and many others.

But if nervous energy should be diminished, which means that there should be a state of enervation, all these essential functions of the organisms will be diminished as well. This is why enervation of the organism leads to a slow down of elimination, whose function is carried out by the kidneys, lungs, cells, etc.

Let's take exposure to cold, for example. It always enervates the organism. Thus, the organs of eliminations and the cells, lacking the flux of abundant energy, slow down their work. The result: increased toxemia and wastes that the body will eliminate in the form of mucus, if the quantity goes above the individual level of toleration.

The Toxemic Level and Variable Tolerance

When a person is perfectly healthy, enervation will not lead to a cold, because it's not enough to elevate toxemia beyond the tolerance level.

We've seen that the common cold and flu will manifest themselves when enervation in the organism will make the waste level overflow, by slowing down elimination. Here, the tolerance level for toxemia lowers by increased toxemia. But this level could also lower (and lead to a cold) through increased individual vitality. In the first case, the body doesn't tolerate the wastes anymore, having reached such a high level. In the second case, even though the wastes could be in small quantity, the body doesn't tolerate them because it has a stronger vitality that no longer accepts this toxemia.

Thus, a person in good health will reject rapidly and violently toxemia with a fever, for example. On the other hand, a weak person of poor health doesn't have the strength to eliminate the wastes. This person will only have a slight fever or none at all. *Acute illnesses belong to the strong and chronic illnesses to the weak.*

In this manner, when we go on vacation, take extra rest, and increase vitality, a cold could manifest itself. The stronger health is the less it will tolerate toxemia and the more it will react against it. It's the same when we change our diet for a healthier one. The vital forces will increase after a while and proceed to clean out wastes they use to tolerate before but no longer do because they now have the strength and power to eliminate them. Disease is elimination.

Finally, when we fast, the forces of the body are liberated of the tiresome work of digestion and turn towards the work of elimination. The person fasting might become sick to actively eliminate.

(Note by F.P: This last part by Mosséri is essential to understand. It also goes in hand with the Law of Vital Accommodation that I presented in my book the *Raw Secrets*. A healthy person will not tolerate even the smallest amount of toxin, while an unhealthy person could eat donuts and drink coffee all day and not notice a difference. But the unhealthy person is slowly marching towards a state of chronic illness while the healthy person is keeping their body clean and avoiding the prospect of chronic illness).

What About Sick People?

Sick people must take drugs, right?

You, as the reader of those innocent lines, yes you, and not somebody else, will you please be able to tell us why do we think that only sick people - and not healthy people - must take medication?

I have not found the answer to this embarrassing question, and I truly hope that a discerning reader would be kind enough to explain to me the reason why, presuming that he would have been able to solve this impossible problem first.

While waiting for your guidance, I maintain that healthy and sick people need the same essential substances. I also maintain what the harmful substances are the same for everybody.

So if there is a food or drug that is essential to a category of people, then it must be essential to all of us, even to the sick people.

To recap:

1. Certain unhealthy habits, mostly in diet, lower nervous energy of the body (enervation).

2. This enervation slows down elimination.

3. This slowing down of elimination increases the level of toxemia.

4. When toxemia reaches the level of tolerance— slowly or abruptly—and goes beyond it, a crisis of elimination (disease) will manifest itself to eliminate this excess.

5. This crisis will take the form of an acute or chronic illness.

Sublata Causa, Tollitur Effectus.

```
(Note by FP: This previous title is in Latin and means: the
effect ceases when the cause is removed.)
```

We've seen that disease is a beneficial elimination, and that it's harmful to fight it. "Almost all men die from their remedies and not from their diseases."—Molière

It would then be advisable to address the causes instead of vainly addressing the effects (the symptoms). The common cold is a process of compensatory elimination that the body establishes to eliminate its internal "dirt," along with its symptoms, as soon as the toxemia level lowers below the level of toleration. And this happens with whatever treatment, and even more rapidly, without any treatment!

This is why any remedy appears to cure the common cold. We then attribute the "cure" to the last treatment. And why not to the treatment before that last one? And why not in spite of all these treatments?

Natural Hygiene Is Not Therapy

Natural Hygiene is not a healing art — it is not a therapy.

We consider diseases as the result of an abuse of the physiological laws. The one and only condition to heal is to follow Nature's Law.

What is the purpose of animal and human experimentation? This medical research is useless and leads nowhere.

What is disease? As we just said, this is an elimination process.

Examples:

- cold, bronchitis and sinusitis cause catarrhs eliminating toxins;
- diarrhea eliminates putrid matter;
- fever burns and eliminates the acidifying wastes of the metabolism;
- cough eliminates sputum containing toxins.

Diseases are Nature's way to purify, repair and rejuvenate the organism. We should not fight against diseases.

Diseases are never harmful, if you let them take their course, without counterattacking with poisons or other so-called natural means. Fever is never dangerous if you stay warm, bedridden and not eating any food. Nature's processes are not dangerous. Their purpose is to palliate to the unhealthy conditions the patient is stuck in. The danger comes when people try to relieve fever.

People are not killed by disease, but by treatments, as said Moliere in a similar way.

Medicine keeps fighting symptoms, instead of fighting their causes that are artificial food, coffee, tobacco, chocolate, wine, etc.

The Healing Power

Here is a question I am often asked:

- Do healing substances exist?
- Not at all, would I categorically reply. Only living matter – plant or animal - may have a healing ability.

The ability to heal itself without external assistance is the cell's inherent capability.

A cut would heal even on a plant, but not on a stone.

The healing power cannot be transferred from a person to another, like from a healer to his patient. This is a personal capability that only cells have.

Healing Is Not Immediate

Recovery and healing are not immediate. These are ongoing processes —like life—evolving in a very strict way and requiring some time.

Moreover, these processes require growth materials and energy influx as well as cellular nutrition and elimination.

No substance can help with the healing process if it is not a substance that is naturally related to the organism and is essential to life.

All the healing agents are naturally and physiologically related to our biology. They can be used in a constructive way to reinforce health, to heal or to recover health.

As an example, bricks may be used to build a house, but the same bricks must be used to repair the house.

How to Dose Hygiene Factors

While medicine prescribes useless and harmful poisons (drugs), Natural Hygiene recommends hygienic factors (food, physical activity, rest) according to the patient's needs.

Indeed, a patient will not require the same amount of food, sleep, physical activity, and sun than a healthy person. This is where lays all the professional Natural Hygiene ability, experience, and sensitivity in treating patients.

Nature's Law Cannot Be Violated Without Any Consequences

Medicine offers remedies to avoid the inevitable consequences of an unhealthy lifestyle. This is simply not possible. Just the thought of it is immoral. Nature's Law and Life's Laws cannot be violated without any consequences.

Remedies are deceptive: in the best case they mask the symptoms for some time. But these symptoms always reappear under a different form, because once the organism starts to recover, it will try again to eliminate the poisons.

People then keep on using the remedy thinking it is the right thing to do but this causes a total degeneration of the organism, that eventually collapses.

Let's consider heartburn. The doctor will prescribe a drug to neutralize this inconvenient pain. The person does not feel any pain anymore and is happy with the situation.

Alas, even if the damages are not obvious, even if the person does not feel any pain anymore, the trouble remains, hidden under the appearance of a false kidney pain or headache or somewhere else in the body. Kidneys also have to eliminate this alkaline remedy. Instead of having just one disease we end up with two!

Hiding Under Technical Vocabulary

In order to hide the nonsense of medicine, a highly medical, technical, obscure lingo is used, as well as complicated and mysterious sentences and wording.

Medical students and the general public are forced to make a huge effort to understand this very complicated language, and that prevents them from having a rational thinking. Nicolas Boileau-Despréaux said in similar terms, "Whatever is well conceived is clearly said... and the words to say it flow with ease." That means that what is not easy to conceive will come in a very obscure way. This is what happens with medicine.

The entire *materia medica* (the study of drugs) is lacking rationality. Hence, the utilization of highly complicated terms mask the knowledge deficiency and prevent people from thinking.

Is it normal to teach people that Nature's Law may be violated?

How is it possible to balance the consequences of an unhealthy lifestyle that goes against Nature's laws without trying to make it healthier? With remedies?

Let's be serious. Nature did not provide humans with remedies, but with punishment in the form of diseases and healing crisis.

The one and only way to heal is to eliminate the cause. When the cause is removed, the consequences disappear.

However, it is not easy for the patient to find the different causes of his troubles by himself. There are primary and secondary causes. An effort that does not address the right cause may be very deceptive.

As an example, there is no point to address secondary causes if you have not previously dealt with primary causes. At first, it is best not to bother with secondary causes. Only a professional natural hygienist will be able to guide you.

It is best to look at how medicine is effective before examining the effectiveness of Natural Hygiene. Modern medicine is a total failure: public health degenerates day after day, the number of patients keeps on increasing. There are now millions of people suffering from cancer, even babies — who used to be disease-free — are also afflicted. Hospitals are full with patients and cannot deal with all of them.

When it is said there is "medical progress," it is to dissimulate this total failure. Treating the causes did not make a lot of progress. On the other hand, surgery did.

There is another phenomenon. Thousands of people who were left aside by modern medicine as incurable, moved to Natural Hygiene and, amazingly, got back on their feet. This includes people suffering from asthma, mental disorders, heart disease, benign cancer, psoriasis, eczema, headaches lasting for 30 years, sterility, herpes, eye infections, insomnia, arthritis, gangrene, and many more.

Final Notes to This Chapter by Frederic Patenaude

With this exposé by Mosséri on the nature of disease, I know a lot of questions are left out. Are all diseases "eliminations"? What about cancer?

Some people might also be wondering if this explanation of disease might not be too simplistic.

With all of the knowledge we have about virology and immunity, it seems to be overly primitive to qualify all diseases as "elimination crisis."

Natural Hygiene presents a model of disease and health that in most cases, can work a lot better than the traditional model. When Natural Hygiene was "invented," doctors were treating their patients with toxic remedies that often killed them, and telling them they should not bathe more than once a month.

We now know for sure that some diseases are indeed transmittable. But even with that in mind, the concept of toxemia is still valuable.

More research definitely needs to be done to bring Natural Hygienic principles in line with current scientific knowledge.

Robert Koch, the same man who discovered the bacteria causing tuberculosis, established four criteria designed to establish a clear relationship between cause and effect from microbes to disease. These criteria are commonly referred to as "Koch's Postulates," which are:

1. The microorganism must be found in abundance in all organisms suffering from the disease, but should not be found in healthy animals.
2. The microorganism must be isolated from a diseased organism and grown in pure culture.
3. The cultured microorganism should cause disease when introduced into a healthy organism.
4. The microorganism must be re-isolated/isolated from the inoculated, diseased experimental host and identified as being identical to the original specific causative agent.

Nowadays, these postulates have a more historical importance. Many agents accepted as causing specific diseases do not fulfill all of Koch's postulates. I nonetheless bring up these postulates in order to put in perspective what we've learned from Mosséri in this chapter.

The notion of toxemia has not been accepted by mainstream medicine. But who said that mainstream medicine was after health and not just elimination of symptoms? Natural Hygiene is after health, recognizes that only elements essential to life can bring about true health, and that the primary action needed for restoring health is the elimination of the causes of illness.

But even mainstream medicine now accepts the fact that at least 75% of all diseases are diet and lifestyle related.

Mainstream medicine also admits that there is no cure for the common cold.

This is where the toxemia concept—although not perfect—it can nonetheless help you lead a healthier life.

Addressing the *cause* of a health problem will always lead to better results than ignoring it.

Keep in mind that most of Mosséri's patients came to him as a *last resort* when modern medicine failed them.

That being said, there are quite a few instances where drugs, such as antibiotics, and surgery, can save your life. I urge you to keep in mind the context in which Mosséri wrote those lines. When in doubt, I always suggest consulting medical doctors that also have a training in Natural Hygiene, such as the excellent staff of the *True North Health Center* in California.

Made in the USA
San Bernardino, CA
09 August 2017